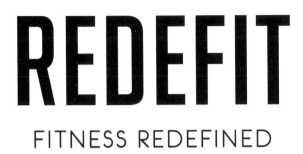

REDEFIT

FITNESS REDEFINED

Scott Schutte, Nate Kesterson & Janine Stichter, Ph.D.

CONTENTS

RedeFit - Fitness Redefined

It's time to look at fitness through a different lens.

PREFACE

The RedeFit Model is our revolutionary approach to health and fitness. Through this program we are redefining fitness by taking a holistic approach. We want to make sure that no part of you is left behind as you move toward the lean, healthy, and happy life you've always wanted. As complex human beings, we are more than our bodies, minds, and environment alone. Our uniqueness comes from the combination of all three. All too often, other health and fitness programs target single aspects of our lives and as a result, many of us do not see the long-term outcomes we desire.

The RedeFit Model will give you hope again and show you that the seemingly impossible is possible. This book contains the tools to achieve and sustain your fitness goals. A leaner, healthier, happier you awaits!

Let's take a quick peek at what is in store for you on your RedeFit journey. The first three chapters are designed to provide you with an overview of why we believe the fitness industry needs an update and what that should look like. Chapter 1 shows how the current approach has failed. In Chapter 2 we explain the importance of redefining fitness in becoming lean, healthy and happy. Chapter 3 presents the details of the RedeFit Model.

The remaining chapters provide insight on each of 10 unique areas that we feel are essential to consider in any effective approach to fitness. Chapter 4 shows you the important role mindset plays in how you view the world, your life, and your fitness; we give you steps to take right away to improve your mindset. Chapter 5 offers innovative approaches for managing your stress. Chapter 6 dispels misconceptions about happiness and helps you determine what happiness looks like for you. In Chapter 7 we examine how relationships influence your stress, happiness, and fitness levels and give you practical approaches for improving them. In Chapter 8 we help you see nutrition as one of your most powerful tools in achieving the look, vitality, and health you desire. In Chapter 9 we present proactive and accessible steps for improving your health. Chapter 10 focuses on the physical elements of your RedeFit journey—stamina, flexibility, and strength—and presents recommendations for achieving a balance for a long-lasting, healthy, and active life. And in Chapter 11 you will learn that by becoming leaner, healthier, and happier, you can influence and inspire the people around you through a practice we call *Giving Fit Back*. Are you ready for your unique RedeFit journey that will change your life?

The model we've developed for this book is a multi-dimensional approach that reflects our collaboration. This book is a product of the combined efforts of three professionals with backgrounds in health, nutrition, fitness, and behavioral psychology. Scott Schutte and Nate Kesterson have spent the last 12 years learning from and working with the best of the best in the health and fitness industry to identify the optimal practices in helping clients achieve their goals. These professionals have included traditional medical doctors, functional medical doctors, Chinese medical doctors, PhDs, psychologists, physical therapists, strength coaches, personal trainers, yoga instructors, life coaches, and chiropractors to improve people's health and fitness. They co-founded and built the highly successful fitness center Columbia Strength & Conditioning. Since 2010 they have been managing a team of trainers and have worked with thousands of clients to refine the Redefit Model.

Dr. Janine Stichter is a behaviorist who has been helping individuals and organizations create positive behavior change for two decades, both as a researcher and clinician. She has conducted over 100 national and international presentations, has written over 90 peer-reviewed research papers, and has contributed to numerous books. With a Ph.D. in behavior analysis, she understands the complexity of behavior and the need for a multi-faceted lifestyle approach for sustained change.

Chapter 1

The Broken Fitness Industry

It's time to look at fitness through a different lens.

If you're reading *RedeFit*, this probably isn't your first time trying to get fit. You have likely tried and have been disappointed at least once on this journey, probably many times. We want to let you in on a secret. You didn't fail; the fitness industry—the diet and exercise programs—you counted on to deliver results failed you. Despite the multi-billion-dollar industry and corresponding diets, there are more obesity-related health issues than ever before. Three out of four people in the United States are overweight. One in three is not just overweight but obese. You read that right— nearly 75% of the U.S. population is overweight and over a third are obese. Clearly, the system has failed you and those around you. The market is flooded with nutrition and fitness advice, with extremes like significant calorie reduction, highly restricted food intake, unrealistic training demands, or programs that urge you to break from family and friends, so you can devote your days to workouts and nutrition.

So, why do most people fail to reach or maintain their fitness goals? What's wrong with the current approach so many people take? It comes down to this: setting the wrong goals and taking the wrong path. Failure often springs from not properly defining the appropriate goal and then using misguided strategies to achieve it.

Let's look at some examples that will resonate with you to illustrate this. Take "Susan." Her primary goal is weight loss and her strategy is massive calorie reduction. This is a very common and very unsuccessful scenario. Why might this be the wrong goal for Susan? Although excess weight can contribute to health-related issues, so can many other things such as stress and sleep deprivation. Admittedly, if Susan can maintain her self-imposed deprivation for two weeks, she will lose weight. But is that the end goal she really seeks? Will her health suffer? Will she feel good, look good, have energy, and be someone people want to be around? Not likely. She will be grumpy, cognitively slow, and have low energy. Yes, she might be able to fit into her skinny jeans, but at what cost and for how long?

And what about Susan's choice of significant caloric restriction as a strategy? Massively slashing calories is a short-term solution that achieves short-term results. In fact, people who do this often experience the yo-yo effect—they alternate between weight loss and weight gain, but they are never stable. If weight loss were easily accomplished by dramatically reducing calories and this approach was sustainable over time, why are most Americans overweight? Calorie restriction is difficult to calculate, extreme calorie deficits are hard to maintain in the long-term, and this method only addresses part of the problem.

So, what is the solution? *Redefine it.* Clarify what Susan really needs and what she is lacking. If Susan is unhappy at work, has parents in poor health, and has children that require a lot of attention, the last thing she needs is to further deprive herself by cutting to extremely low calories. Changing Susan's diet will take discipline and urging her to become more disciplined during a stressful time in her life is not the best approach. And it won't stick. When people are overwhelmed or emotionally drained, the focus should be replenishing their well-being and sense of self. Therefore, the initial focus must be more balanced. To achieve well-being, Susan needs help managing her stress. When cortisol levels or other stress hormones are high, it is difficult to stick to an exercise plan or stay away from unhealthy snacks which will make it almost impossible to lose weight and feel better. Instead, we can increase Susan's fun, improve her sleep, increase her connections, and enrich her purpose?

Susan is not alone in her singular approach to becoming fitter and leaner. Let's look at another example that we often see—a client approaching us with the goal of getting fit by running a marathon. "Emily" had the goal to get in shape and decided to train for a marathon as her strategy. Now, if Emily has had running experience, loves to run, and a marathon has long been her dream, then we fully support her goal. But, if a marathon is something she just picked as her journey to getting fit, we have some concerns. The amount of time, as well as physical and mental stress her body must endure in training for a marathon, might actually make her less fit. Running a long distance doesn't make a person fit; it may not even make them good at running. The goal of being fit needs to include feeling good, moving well, and increased happiness, but someone training to run long distances alone will not do the trick.

The solution is to *redefine it* and to clarify what Emily really needs and what she is lacking. After several conversations with Emily, we learned that she really enjoyed being part of her high school track team and is looking to create connections like those she had in high school. Emily already runs several times a week but repeatedly injures herself before she works up to the mileage required for a marathon.

There are two paths for helping Emily. She could continue her marathon training and add strength and flexibility training. This will help her body withstand the mileage of marathon training and help her recover and move more efficiently. Another option could be for Emily to meet her need for connection by building friendships in the running community and even ask her running friends to do strength and flexibility training with her. If connection through fitness is her ultimate goal, she can exchange the grueling and time-consuming marathon goal for running shorter distances with a running club and partnering with friends to enhance strength and prevent injuries. She can achieve her goal with less time invested and reduced injuries.

Let's look at one more example. "Mike" wants to get below 10 percent body fat, and his strategy to getting there is to work out extremely hard five days a week. Despite his efforts in the gym, he still can't get there. Why might this strategy not be working for him? The problem is no matter how hard Mike works out, his food choices are not serving him, so he struggles to lose body fat. What should Mike do?

Once again, the solution is to *redefine it*; to clarify what Mike needs and what he is lacking. Mike has a close relationship with his children. However, as they get older, they are becoming more involved in sports and he recognizes that his happiness is enhanced by being able to participate. Mike's obstacle is that he eats out on the weekends (which makes it easy to overeat) and after 15 years of this lifestyle choice, he is 30 pounds overweight. He needs to work on healthier choices when eating out and stop eating out as much. We will see some impact on his body fat loss with these initial steps, but the likelihood that we are going to hit sub-10 percent is low. Can Mike get to sub-10 percent body fat? Maybe, but it will require some trade-offs. Perhaps he can prepare food at home, so he knows the ingredients that are going into his meals. Sure, he will be eating healthier, but he won't be eating out with his family anymore. He will become leaner, but it will also isolate him from his family and add stress to his busy life. Is that helping him achieve his goal of enhancing his happiness through interactions with his children? Maybe achieving sub-10 percent body fat isn't the right goal for Mike. After conversations with Mike, we determined that he wanted to spend lots of time with his children, so we worked with him on carefully choosing healthy items when eating out and encouraged him to cook meals at home with his children. Both approaches will contribute to his happiness.

We're not saying you should not try to lose body fat, get to a healthy weight, or run. We are saying that dramatic lifestyle changes might not be the best solution for your actual goals, desires, and long-term success. First, identify what you really need, set the right goals, and then start on the path to achieving them. That's why we wrote this book.

This book is not about going to extremes in the area of well-being or health; it's about making a balanced, focused impact on your overall fitness in order to reach your personal goals and desired lifestyle. It's about finding the areas you are passionate about for your fitness and creating sustained change in those areas to reach your personal goals and desired lifestyle. And more importantly, it provides a process that you can use as those passions shift and evolve for a sustainable lifestyle.

But this need for a new approach extends beyond you and into your inner circle. This system that's failing you is also failing those close to you.

Like it or not, you're an influencer and the people you choose to be around influence you. The actions, the examples, the very person you are influences those around you. And probably more than you think, especially if you have children or if children are a regular part of your life. Little ones soak up everything around them, regardless of its intent or effect. It has been said that each of us is a composite of the five people we spend the most time with. This effect extends to income, happiness, occupation, and, yes, weight and health. Now, this doesn't necessarily mean you should walk up to your overweight friends and say, "Sorry, we can't hang out anymore. You're a negative influence." Influencing is a two-way street. Instead, it means taking the reins and realizing that it's part of our responsibility as their friend to inspire them and influence them to improve their life.

Believe it or not, you're influencing and leading more people than you know. You've achieved near super-hero status in terms of the power you're wielding, not only to help shape others in a positive direction but to steer your own life.

You have the power to create an environment that elevates you and the five people closest to you. However, to break free from the norms—to leave the super-majority—takes courage. There is short-term comfort in staying with the average, sticking with the norm. But you're reading this book because you want more.

This book will provide you with the tools and strategies you need to progress toward a lean, healthy, and happy life. In doing so, you'll be a walking example of success and inspire others to make progress. The progress of those close to you will inspire you to progress even further, which will, in turn, inspire those around you. It's a beautiful virtuous cycle.

The failure of the system and your near super-hero power to impact others are enough to justify the need for this book. You deserve a lean, healthy, and happy life. Until now, you've lacked the right approach for achieving it.

This is where our approach to redefining fitness comes into play. We've created a system to help you find your balance, discover accurate goals for you, and map your optimal path. The tools contained within the following pages are not a blanket prescription; in other words, they are not a set script that applies to everyone. That approach has been done to death and has failed. This book treats you like the unique person you are. It is the key to unlocking your path to well-being. This new approach tailors a path specifically for you. It gives you the tools you need to succeed in your unique place on the lean-healthy-happy spectrum.

Think of your fitness like spokes on a wheel. If any spokes are missing, the wheel can't function at its optimal level. There are ten major spokes in this book on which you will be assessed and have the opportunity to impact. These spokes are: Mindset, Stress Management, Happiness, Relationships, Nutrition, Health, Strength, Stamina, Flexibility, and Giving Fit Back.

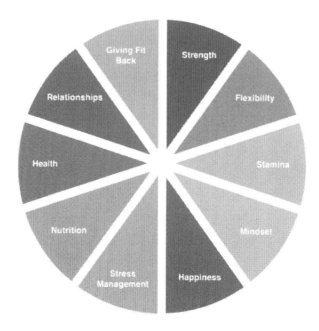

Broken down further, we will consider two main categories:

- The physical side of fitness which includes strength, stamina, and flexibility
- The lifestyle side of fitness which includes nutrition, health, mindset, happiness, stress management, and giving fit back

This book will not only allow you to assess your current state of fitness, health, and well-being, it will also give you the opportunity to set goals with approaches for achieving those goals. Our *Notes from the Doc* feature will further refine the strategies for reframing your thinking and cutting-edge take-home approaches you can start using right away. Let's get started.

NOTES FROM THE DOC

Let me open by saying how excited I am to be one of your guides on this journey. I'm passionate about using my expertise and experience to positively impact people just like you. Frequently the myriad of fitness information is either too vague, too specific, or simply not supported by science. This includes strategies not tailored to you and that, if implemented, would consume huge amounts your time and add to the complexity of your already full schedule. Who can really execute those kinds of plans? Maybe if we could pause all our other responsibilities, we might have a fighting chance. For most of us, that is unrealistic. And even if it were, could we sustain it? Typically, when we put significant time and money into something, we expect significant value in return. Why should we expect anything less for our health and well-being? If you are going to devote time and energy to you, the strategies need to adapt with you, speak to your strengths, evolve with your life and challenge you in ways that you can truly be proud of. Most importantly, they need to be something you can celebrate.

As an expert in behavior change, I have a clear understanding of what it takes to make those initial changes and—this is crucial— sustain those changes. I have had the pleasure of helping people do just that for over 20 years. However, I have not only coached this, I have lived it; I understand the fear, anxiety, frustration, exhilaration, excitement, and freedom that these changes bring.

Due to a medical condition, I gained and lost 70 pounds with each pregnancy. I have raised three children while working full time and helping my husband start his new business. I am now having to learn new things about my body as it matures. Needless to say, I juggle multiple roles, sometimes wearing several hats at once, just like you. I also understand that being lean, healthy, and happy support my roles and amplifies the impact I have on my loved ones. By using targeted strategies and having great people beside me along the way, I understand the importance of not jumping from one strategy or quick fix to another. Instead, I take new information and insights and pair them with the behaviors already in place and adjust. This has created opportunities for small corrections without getting caught up in an endless cycle of fads or quick fixes.

Identify and celebrate the success of now. The research is clear. If we want positive results, we must be positive.

You and I have many of the same obstacles and barriers. We're both pursuing the same lean, healthy, and happy lifestyle. In this book, I share scientifically-proven steps that you can realistically follow to help you achieve your goals. You'll find these strategies woven throughout this book and often explored more fully in the *Notes from the Doc* section of each chapter. There, I will share specific ideas, understandings, and strategies to help you succeed.

Let's get started. To be successful and achieve lasting results, we must tackle fundamental behaviors together. This book will provide you with guidance and tools you can start using right away. But first, we need to set the foundation, so you can access and be successful with these resources. In other words, I want to tip the scales in your favor through science.

----

*Research across many disciplines indicates that we need a ratio
of four positive words to counteract every negative one.*

STAYING POSITIVE

Identify and celebrate the success of now. The research is clear.
If we want to increase our chances for success, we must be positive. We begin by recognizing what we currently have. It may
be your attitude toward others, a favorite body part, a behavior
change made in the past that you still maintain, or your relationships. Openly identify and acknowledge them. Trust me, it will
make your future obstacles smaller, and it will accelerate you on
your journey. This is not just a feel-good mantra; this has been
studied for over 100 years. The research has investigated the impact of mental thoughts on physical movement (think: sports psychology) as well as how positive words can impact our cognitive
reasoning, accessing and prompting into action our motivation
centers. Conversely, negative words access our sense of fear, releas-
ing corresponding hormones and impacting our reasoning, mo-
tor skills, response time and overall functioning. For example, a
recent study from Harvard Business School[1] looked at the impact
of affirmative language on anxiety. Participants who felt anxious
prior to activities such a public speaking or singing were asked
to engage in altered self-talk. As opposed to just trying to "calm
down" (which is difficult and often ineffective to do with the high
levels of physiological arousal that accompany anxiety) they were
told to tell themselves that they were "excited" to do the activity.
This is called reappraisal of an emotion, anxious is reappraised as

excitement as opposed to suppression, anxiousness is hidden to appear calm. Because both anxiety and excitement have similar physiological symptoms (i.e, increased heart rate) it is much easier on the body and cognitive load to make this mindset shift. The results of several studies indicate that reappraisal to a positive action or state improves performance and self-efficacy about the task[2]. And, because we are prewired for self-preservation, we respond to negative words much more than positive ones. Research across many disciplines indicates that to make positive change we need a minimum of four positive words to for every negative one. It provides the necessary specific feedback to our brains of the behaviors that are working and need to be repeated, as opposed to focusing on what has not worked. Studies in education, business, and relationships highlighted the significant importance of this ratio for learning, effective business teams, and successful marriages. It is what our brains need to process and act on the positive. As an example: although I might be frustrated that I overslept and missed my morning workout, I should highlight that I did set my alarm to work out, that I did buy healthy food to take for lunch, and that I have plans to walk with a co-worker during break. All too often, once we have that initial set-back we continue our pattern of negative talk that sabotages any further attempts for success towards our goals that day. So, can you see how this is critical to your success on this journey? It's not an easy change, but it's one you must buy into from the start.

Here are some easy-to-use approaches to start right away: ask like-minded positive friends and family to hold you accountable, talk to yourself in the car, and catch yourself before you get attached to a negative thought or belief. Lastly, set an initial goal of saying at least three more positive than negative things about yourself each day. These do not have to be complicated self-affirming conversations. Simply recognize the things like the reps, steps, sleep, and good nutrition choices you made, no matter how small. Even if your schedule only allows a brief moment, take that time to begin practicing positivity. It will propel you forward.

A key tenet of Malcolm Gladwell's book, *Outliers,* is that those who are extraordinary put in countless hours of focused practice. An important note: it was not extensive focus on everything in their life, but on a few key areas they were passionate about. This book is not about being an outlier in the area of health or well-being; it's about making a focused impact on your overall fitness to reach your personal goals and desired lifestyle. As we have already illustrated, the fitness industry is full of either hyper-focused approaches, such as a fad diets, or programs that seemingly encourage you to disown family and friends and quit your job so you can devote all your time to perfectly planning your day, workouts and nutrition. Of course, none of it is realistic. In isolation, these practices often lack key steps that science has shown necessary for effective and long-lasting behavior change. So, where do we begin to change our journey? Let's start with focus.

THE IMPORTANCE OF PRIORITIES

Where are your greatest pain points? You might like to adjust, improve, or optimize many things, but what are the few, the priority areas, that you really need to overhaul? Why is it so important to identify priorities? Behavior change must be acknowledged and celebrated by the person making the change. For example, recovering alcoholics count each day of sobriety and celebrate annual anniversaries. This consistent recognition and celebration help form new habits. You might be thinking correctly that alcohol is an addiction, and you don't have an addiction; you just want to change a few things. But consider how long you have you been doing those things. Do you not consider chronic stress an addiction? You know that you should say "no" to more requests and set parameters on your valuable time. If you know this, why don't you do it? Have you tried and failed? Perhaps you enjoy crossing things off your to-do list, showing people you can handle it. This constant cycle creates a chemical response in your brain that contributes to a feedback loop of doing and craving more.

Let's return to the alcoholic. She has a failing marriage, poor health, and her job is at risk. What is her most critical need here? Curtailing or giving up drinking, of course. To that end, she gets support through coaching and replaces drinking with fitness activities to improve her health. This allows her to spend more quality time on her marriage and improve her attendance and work performance—all desired changes. Coaching helps her focus on the key priorities that will best enable her to form new habits. This provides the greatest return on her investment because when we tackle too much, we dilute our efforts and results.

Now replace alcohol with stress. When your stress is high, it negatively impacts your health and reduces opportunities for quality time with friends and family. Anyone who has endured high levels of stress knows that ignoring it and trying to have a little downtime or fun is short-lived. Why? Because the need to resolve the stress and its overall health impact takes its toll. Once again, the priority should be to identify stress triggers and lasting solutions.

Reducing stress-generated cortisol is key to long-lasting impact on the other aspects of your life.

Another very important aspect of identifying and addressing the priority areas first is the increased ability to measure and celebrate progress. Everyone has heard the expression: the last five pounds are the hardest to lose. Aside from the physiological reasons for this, one key reason is that it's harder to see and feel the incremental changes over a month or two. At best, we are talking just ounces a week. How will you measure and celebrate incremental progress toward addressing your focus?

Priorities are ever-changing depending on your life circumstances, such as moving up the career ladder, having a new family, dealing with aging parents, or encountering financial challenges. And, somehow, as life events and circumstances evolve, we never seem to gain any more time. Let's work smarter, not harder. We do not have time to try every new idea, diet, or behavior change program. We need a system customized for us that accesses the skillsets we have developed to address priorities as they come and go in our lives.

We are thrilled to share our expertise with you and help you on your path to fitness. Allow us to do the heavy lifting in integrating the complexity as you read this book, identify your key priorities and engage on this exciting journey.

CHAPTER 2
CREATING A HABIT OF CONSISTENCY

"We're drowning in information while starving for wisdom."
–E.O. Wilson

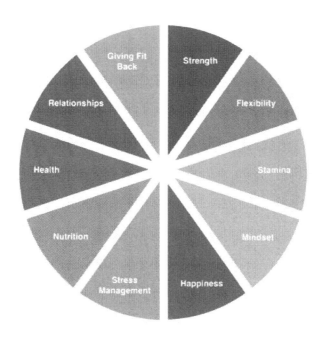

MAKING SENSE OF THE FITNESS INFORMATION OVERLOAD

In order to begin your fitness journey, you must know where to start. That's a challenge in today's world; information is every-where. One of the problems with having access to so much health and fitness information is making sense of conflicting messages. In the world of fitness, the pendulum constantly swings from one extreme to the other. Some experts claim that without question the low-fat approach is healthiest. Then other experts say no, actu-ally high-fat is best. When it comes to losing weight, we hear that cardio gets the best results and, on the other hand, we hear that strength training does. Heck, even something as simple as break-fast isn't even straightforward. Some claim it is the most impor-tant meal of the day while others assert that skipping breakfast will burn more fat and improve your health. When the experts can't agree on something as simple as breakfast, what are we sup-posed to do? And then there's the sensationalism as every week ushers in a new fad or acronym, each claiming to be better than the last one and easier to follow—the ketogenic diet (keto); high-intensity interval training (HIIT); the carnivore diet; the paleo diet; intermittent fasting; the raw food diet; time-restricted eat-ing; juice cleanses; calories in, calories out (CICO); if it fits your macros (IIFYM), and whatever new one is hot right now. It's enough to make your head spin. With so much health and fitness information out there, it's challenging to know which direction to take in your health and fitness journey. This uncertainty can lead to inaction or ineffective action, neither of which will get you to your goals.

In defense of the wealth of the information available, fitness can be very difficult to study. And the studies aren't typically funded unless someone can profit from the outcome. Other challenges include factoring in genetics, health history, and environment while also convincing a group to follow a plan accurately and consistently for a long period of time. With these limitations, there is much confusion, many conflicting theories, and a lot of noise. The answer to this noise is a different way to view the information and your approach. But, as we dive deeper, you will see it's not the lack of quality information that holds people back but setting the right goals and keeping one's path simple that are the keys to success.

To make an analogy, think of all the fitness information and recommendations as shoes. Yes, shoes. Countless studies and different approaches can provide some direction, but this information is analogous to having more choices in footwear. You would like shoes that fit and are appropriate for the occasion: dress shoes for a business environment or sneakers for the gym but definitely not high heels for a half-marathon (ouch!). Having access to so many types of footwear enables you to match the appropriate shoe to the occasion. Like the shoes, we want to apply the same criteria to health and fitness information. Does it fit you and is the information appropriate in each situation?

So, when it comes to low fat vs. high fat, cardio or strength training, breakfast or intermittent fasting, or any of the other choices before us, we need to identify the right approach at the right time for the proper goal. We need to pick the appropriate "shoe." For some, cardio training is a more appropriate "shoe" at that time than resistance training. For some others, it's the other way around. How do we know when it's the right choice? That depends on the person, namely you. And as the saying goes: if the shoe fits, wear it. You need a tailored approach and that's the beauty of this book. It will be customized to you based on the person that knows you best: you.

You'll assemble the information needed to decide when it's time to use a particular "shoe" based on your goals, current situation, and schedule. You'll finally be able to cut through the confusion and bring certainty to your fitness journey.

It's liberating to know that you're on the right path—that your search for a plan customized to you has ended. You can relax knowing that you've found what you've been looking for. With some of the external factors addressed, it's time to turn inward and to examine your identity and the phase of your unique journey.

It's not the lack of quality information that holds people back but setting the right goals and keeping one's path simple that are the keys to success.

HOW DOES IDENTITY AFFECT YOUR HEALTH?

When you consider that billions of dollars spent on fitness, that there's a fitness facility or coach on every corner, and that one of the top New Year's resolutions is getting fit, why do so many people struggle to reach their fitness goals? Is there a lack of incentive to do what it takes to become fit? Is there a lack of knowledge? Is it because their identity is tied to unhealthy habits? Let's dig into this.

Your Identity and Your Environment

Your identity affects your behaviors and opportunities. Even minute shifts in our perception of ourselves or others' perceptions of us dramatically affect our actions and our options. Let's look at an example of the power of identity to shape behavior.

Sophia is by all standards, a healthy and fit woman. If she is perceived as a fit person at work, she is less likely to bring junk food to the office. There is less chance she'll be offered the leftover cake at the office party. There is a greater chance Sophia will be invited to join a coworker for a run. But if Sophia has a different identity, say, for example, one of being a talented baker, then she might be more likely to bring cookies to share with coworkers and they will bring her treats in return. As a person who enjoys sweets, Sophia is more likely to be asked to go for ice cream at the new gelato place after work, and less likely to be invited to go work out with a coworker.

This may seem like a minor thing, but over time your identity plays a big role in your daily activities. These identities might have little to do with your true personality; you might love to run but also bake great cookies. Once you have an identity within a circle of people, it is difficult to change. Think about ways the people in your circles perceive you and expect you to behave. How can you shape an identity that will enable you to be viewed as your ideal healthy self, helping you on your journey to becoming your best self?

Your Identity and Your Choices

Often when we are motivated for change, we're simultaneously impatient for results. It is only natural. After all, who doesn't want to reach their goals as soon as possible? But this is where we need to be careful. The temptation to accelerate progress often leads to the treacherous strategy of increasing intensity. For example, instead of simply working on adjusting your daily routines to get your daily activity in—which takes mindfulness and planning—we often see people wake up one morning and decide that they are not only going to get their daily activity in, but they have vowed to sleep eight hours every night, regularly eat a protein-rich breakfast, drink enough water, begin weight training five days a week, and start meditating. You get the point.

Inconsistency leads to stagnation. Stagnation leads to loss of motivation.

We've all been there. The intent is great, but the reality is exhausting and at times deflating. The fatigue and stress that accompany so many major changes lead to inconsistency. Then inconsistency leads to stagnation. Stagnation leads to loss of motivation. And we're right back where we started—or in an even worse predicament.

It's time for a different strategy. We promote the concept of "consistency over intensity"—the practice of adopting a few simple behaviors at a time that are implementable and sustainable for you. Only after you've become proficient with those behaviors do you add more, thereby minimizing the fatigue and stress associated with additional changes. This concept of "consistency over intensity" will be your key to lasting results. Let's consider some real-world examples.

"Even the most tailored plan will fail without embracing the concept of "consistency over intensity." —Notes from the Doc

----

Connor is healthy, works out regularly, eats right, and mostly feels great. One night, Connor goes out drinking with old college friends. He wakes up the next day feeling unmotivated, tired, and lethargic in stark contrast to most mornings. Drinking that night wasn't as fun as in college, and the next day Connor paid the price: he didn't have his normal high level of energy and enthusiasm. Although it was good to see old friends, was it worth wasting the next day? It's easy to make the choice not to do this regularly. This is an example of why fit people tend to stay fit; it is punishing to practice unhealthy behaviors.

Now imagine April, a person who is unhealthy, doesn't work out much, eats poorly, and feels crummy most of the time. After work, April goes out for a healthy dinner with a friend. The food tastes flavorless to her. After the meal, she still feels hungry and unsatisfied. April wonders why anyone would want to lead such a bland life of deprivation. April says, "Life is short; enjoy it!" and her friend wholeheartedly agrees. One healthy meal is not likely to make an unhealthy person feel better and deprives them of their usual immediate gratification from an unhealthy meal. So, the person thinks: *was it worth it?* This is an example of why unfit people tend to stay unfit. It is punishing to practice healthy behaviors in the short-term.

An unhealthy meal can make a healthy person feel bad, and similarly, a healthy meal may not make an unhealthy person feel good. In both cases, each person is reinforced for continuing their habits, but one is helpful, and the other is not. This is a cycle that continues and what makes this even more difficult is as we age, we can't get away with as many unhealthy lifestyle choices. Some unhealthy lifestyle choices we made in the past didn't affect us the way they do now.

Think back to your younger years and how quickly you could recover from a night of drinking, sleep deprivation, or even a hard fall. As we age, we need to be more careful about our unhealthy choices if we want to continue to feel great. What we will see is the weekend warrior or the yo-yo dieter who typically has short-term success at best. The problem with this approach of intensity is that it can lead to injury or burnout due to its extreme nature. Shifting identities will not be an immediate fix, but with consistent behaviors, this can be accomplished within any group.

Your Identity and Your Plan

What's the solution? How can we keep an unhealthy person on a plan long enough that they can start to feel good and become a healthy person who is reinforced for their positive choices? Adherence is the key.

The swinging pendulum gives people in the industry a way to stand out, but it confuses the rest of us. As we will repeatedly say in this book, adherence is a key factor in any diet. Why have we seen someone get great results with a low-fat diet when we've seen another person have great results with a high-fat diet? Because they stuck with the program.

"Science indicates that a positive mindset of accomplishment releases hormones, like dopamine, to your brain. When this occurs with consistency, it rewires your brain to better access successful outcomes. Biologists call this the 'winner effect.'"
–Notes from the Doc

Do you know what most diets have in common? Almost all diets cut out processed foods, junk food, candy, alcohol, and other high-calorie foods. The key to success is to find something manageable that hits all your basic nutritional needs. When it comes to exercise, we also have divergent choices. We have one friend who started running every day and got great results and another friend who started lifting weights daily and had excellent results. Which is the right path? Activity is the key; they both became more active. They each adhered to their plans. Now the question is: are they physically balanced doing just one? Time will tell, but more than likely a combination of the two with some flexibility would work best.

IMMERSION VS. SLOW AND STEADY

What's the solution? How do we find a balance that is right for us? And how can we stay on a plan long enough that we can start to see the benefits and become a healthy person reinforced for our positive choices? Two very different approaches to health and fitness can be effective—immersion or slow and steady. Let's examine each one.

Immersion

We are all familiar with immersion. Immersion is an all-in method that typically requires time away from your everyday life—a complete change in your environment. It's often associated with learning a language quickly. Want to learn French? Go live in France for an extended time. Immerse yourself in the language, its nuances, and applications. Also, since most people are speaking French, you won't have much choice but to learn quickly so you can meet your needs and wants. There really is no other choice, which is good because you're there to expedite language learning.

And when your immersion ends, the behaviors developed during that time naturally fade in the absence of consistent and direct effort. When you leave France after your immersion experience, you retain your French for a time. However, without any targeted changes to your natural environment (i.e. opportunities to practice speaking French) as time marches on, your language fluency fades. Continued practice is required.

The same is true when this approach is applied to your fitness. You could immerse yourself in an extended stay retreat where you would blend meditation, journaling, physical activity, healthy meals, relaxation, fun, and sleep. And, since ice cream and cupcakes wouldn't be on the menu, you'd have few temptations and little chance to deviate from your desired behaviors for a healthier you. You would be surrounded by like-minded people reinforcing your healthy behaviors. This approach is highly effective and can be a wonderful tool.

But, like our example of speaking French, it is incomplete by itself. A fitness retreat can be a great way to experience a new level of health, but it needs to be complemented with a comprehensive plan to sustain those habits once you return to reality. It is easy to execute healthy behaviors in the absence of the real world's less than healthy options and stressors. What we need is an approach to navigate those obstacles in our day to day lives. We'll explore that approach next.

"It is human to sometimes drop the ball, however, without a plan or clear goals, we are wired to revert to the path of least resistance." –Notes from the Doc

----

Slow and Steady

Since most of us have few or no opportunities to immerse, and even those that do often struggle with the maintenance of that experience upon returning to their day to day lives, we need another approach. The other method is slow and steady. As this is the more practical approach, slow and steady will be our focus. With this approach, we identify and apply a few simple strategies at a time to reach our goals—both short-term and long-term. This will lead to longer adherence and success. To stick with our previous language analogy, this would be akin to taking a weekly language course. Sure, you won't become fluent as quickly as with the immersion approach, but you will be able to learn the language in a more practical setting as well as systematically create opportunities to maintain it. Such examples include planning trips to French-speaking areas, starting a French-speaking lunch or dinner group, and finding books and magazines to read in French.

Note how this approach mirrors our earlier discussion of

"consistency over intensity." By adopting a few implementable and sustainable strategies at a time, we create a realistic path to lasting results. That is the beauty of the slow and steady pace.

You likely have some ideas about how to improve your fitness. *Can I exercise more? Can I eat out less or reduce my consumption of junk food? Can I spend time meditating or doing something fun and healthy?* If you answered "yes" to any of these, then you are aware of areas through which you can become more fit. But don't let perfect be the enemy of good. We will never have all the information, and it will never be the perfect time. The key is starting. Even the smallest change or effort is a step in the right direction that will take you through several phases. We will explain how to properly assess your goals and choose the path that enables new lifelong habits in the following chapters. To help you get started with this process, let's explore how you typically have tackled your fitness goals.

WHAT'S YOUR FITNESS PACE?

In our professional experience, we tend to see four typical approaches to tackling any new fitness goal.

All in   Slow & Steady   Maintenance   Screw it

All in is what a typical new client thinks they want. This person is looking for a kick-start, detox, or an all-or-nothing approach. Think of "all in" like going on a lifelong journey to explore the world and you start by sprinting out of the gate. You'll burn out quickly and soon feel ready to quit. The key is to slow down your pace and take manageable and focused steps. You learn more, experience more, and enjoy more. An example would be someone who starts the new year working out every day and mostly eats chicken and broccoli. Two weeks later, having done too much too soon, she jumps to "screw it." Her self-talk is, "This is too hard. I'm sore. I'm sick of eating the same food. Life is short. I want to enjoy it." The all-in approach without some guidelines and programmed ways to back off the intensity is rarely a good idea.

Slow and steady is a phase most people don't think of when they start their fitness journey, but it is one that we recommend as a starting point. It calls for minor weekly changes that result in consistent progress. It's not as exciting as all in, because there are no major noticeable weekly changes, but it's more manageable and it creates healthy lifelong habits. Most importantly, it keeps people from regressing to: screw it. Remember, in this lifelong journey of fitness, we need to create habits that become second nature to us. Extremes rarely become habits for long.

Maintenance allows you to keep the progress you made while taking a little break. This pace is the hardest transition for people because it requires work and no real progress. In maintenance, you must stay disciplined most of the time, but it will allow a little less work. You can back off a little on the intensity but not much. Maintenance is great for holidays, travel, or any other life stressor weighing you down. Again, think of it as a lifelong journey. When you need a little break, you don't stop; you slow down, adjust and figure out how to occasionally get back to slow and steady or enjoy living in maintenance. In maintenance you eat healthily most of the time, you are active every day, you have a well-balanced fit life, but you also occasionally allow yourself to eat a meal that is not particularly healthy. You do so guilt-free and without it affecting your overall fitness. This plan doesn't allow you to return to binge-watching TV and eating whatever you want in six weeks. This is forever. And while forever may sound daunting, the key is making it enjoyable, finding activities you like, and eating food you love. It's the best of both worlds—enjoying life and feeling great!

Don't let perfect be the enemy of good.

Screw it is where most people end up after they go all in. This phase cancels all the work they've put in. Keeping with the life-long journey analogy, think of "screw it" like you've stopped the journey and now you're hitching a ride back to where you started. That may sound easy, but it's draining physically and emotionally because you've been working hard to improve only to go back to the beginning and start over again. There are two keys to staying out of screw it. First, take more manageable steps to stick with slow and steady, and when life gets in the way find a way to maintain the progress you've made.

"Old habits are the Goliath to the David of new habits."
–Notes from the Doc

Is it important to understand that there is a place between all in and all out in your fitness journey. Find a pace you can maintain and stay consistent with. Then, as life happens, know how to adjust up and down so you can keep making progress or enjoy the progress you've made. Ultimately the goal is to get the results you are looking for and living in maintenance. This is where you are lean, healthy, and happy.

NOTES FROM THE DOC

CONSISTENCY OVER INTENSITY

As the saying goes: if at first you don't succeed, try, try, and try again. If you're like most people, you can relate to this proverb, especially as it pertains to health and fitness. The fitness industry has provided countless opportunities to try, try, and try again at our fitness goals. As each new method, opportunity, piece of exercise equipment, or life mantra is shared on TV or social media, we are encouraged to try one more time because the latest craze will be the secret to our success. Of course, you should be persistent and keep working toward your desired outcomes, but with one important caveat—you need to try again differently. What does this mean? Clearly, one way to do this is to find the best approach for you, one that is customized to meet your needs. That is the point of this book. However, even the most tailored plan will fail without embracing the concept of "consistency over intensity."

Let me illustrate what I mean. Have you ever done any of the following: missed a workout, had a meal that was not on your diet plan or forgot to call someone back? If you are human, the answer is undoubtedly yes. In response to these lapses of perfection, did you have any of these thoughts: *Clearly, I do not have any energy; I'll just be a couch potato the rest of the day*; *I might as well eat dessert now and start the diet again tomorrow*, or *he's already mad at me; why bother to respond now?* I'm sure you recognize these responses. Most of us have experienced the "screw it" phase described earlier in this chapter. It is human to sometimes drop the ball, however, without a plan or clear goals, we are wired to revert to the path of least resistance. So, when we drop the ball, research suggests that we will not just leave it on the ground; we will step over it and walk away. The next time we drop it, we will deflate it and stomp on it as we walk away. Why? Because once we have failed at something, our brain becomes more conditioned to anticipate that failure again. In response, we will functionally sabotage ourselves even more the next time.

The good news is we can mitigate this cycle and change the outcome. How? By focusing on the three key factors below:

1) Reframing our setbacks so we can learn from them and address the challenge differently.

2) Establishing consistency through specific, targeted goals.

3) Minimizing our sabotages.

REFRAMING SETBACKS

To reframe your setbacks, you need to maximize what worked and minimize what didn't. For example, let's say you started a new diet plan focused on eating more greens and eliminating processed sugar. You stick with it for three days and then on the fourth, you're tempted by a donut at the office. Rather than characterizing your behavior as "ruining your diet," you identify and celebrate (remember Chapter 1) what you did well: four days of increased greens and reduced processed sugar. Science indicates that a positive mindset of accomplishment releases testosterone and dopamine to your brain. When this occurs with consistency, it rewires your brain to better access successful outcomes. Biologists call this the "winner effect." This phenomenon has been recorded in animal studies showing that predators that won initial battles increased their likelihood for successive dominance when factors such as size and innate skills were controlled. In humans, this has been examined in controlled studies of competition as well as in specific groups such as athletes and stock traders. These studies have shown an increased release of specific hormones, such as testosterone, upon winning a competition, as opposed to cortisol upon defeat. Like with the animal studies, people who won were significantly more likely to win again as opposed to those who initially lost. Brain imaging research has also shown differential responses across brain regions based on positive cues, such as "you won" and negative cues, such as "you lost" during competitive scenarios. The mechanisms involved are complex and not fully understood. Yet the end results are real and significantly impact how we approach our lives and our goals.

This literature, as well as several learning theories, indicates that the opposite of the winner effect occurs when you don't create opportunities for success and hence don't release the winning chemicals. You're probably familiar with the term "yo-yo dieting." This refers to the boomerang effect of having initial success with a nutritional or fitness plan but then seeing the gains disappear and returning to baseline. With an actual yo-yo the further down it travels, the harder you must work to get it back up. Eventually, it doesn't even go back up; rather it just dangles. This is not only frustrating, but this cycle does not stimulate our brains to release any positive chemicals and instead releases more cortisol. So, we more quickly give up when we repeat the same activity the same way, such as: the low-sugar diet didn't work; I am going to try a different one.

SET LONG-TERM GOALS WITH A SERIES OF SHORT-TERM GOALS

The research on the effectiveness of goal setting for behavior change is clear, however, most people find goal setting aversive or are not successful because they set all-or-nothing goals. Two examples are: "I will lose 20 pounds by my high school reunion next month," and "I will start getting more sleep this year." These are great goals, but without clear steps toward those goals and markers to celebrate and adjust, you either succeeded or failed. And if you failed, you did so monumentally by not losing the weight this month or failing to fix your sleep habits. Most problematic is that these goals are set up as a one-and-done. Nowhere in your goal is it clear that you will keep the 20 pounds off. Remember those winner-effect chemicals? They are not just a feel-good infusion; they are associated with cognitive processes. The theory, among others, is that this positive influx of chemicals has been linked with cognition. When it surges upon a win, it promotes learning from the experience, heightens skills, and extends the amount of latent learning between wins. So, in the case of behavior change and associated long-term maintenance of performance changes, it is imperative to make consistent small changes (small wins) over time to develop new habits. As such, if we have a goal per week or per month to adjust our nutrition, or get an extra hour of sleep, we are increasingly likely to achieve those milestones. If we have an off week, we will set our sights on next week's goal and this will send good chemicals to our brain.

PLAN FOR YOUR SABOTAGE

Old habits are the Goliath to the David of new habits. For example, you suspect that watching TV before bed is interfering with your sleep. You have heard the recommendations to read a book or try a relaxation technique before bed. Filled with good intentions, you go to your room to read, but the TV remote tempts you. You need to know this new reading habit is going to work before you consider doing something drastic like removing your TV from your bedroom. You think, *I will just watch for a few minutes.* Then you get pulled into your favorite show and a few minutes becomes an hour. This pattern is frustrating and defeating but not surprising given how long you have been watching TV before bed. For some of you it might be 10, 15, even 30 years. Reading for 30 minutes before bed every night for a week may not guarantee that you will not revert to TV watching. Instead, create small goals: read for 5 minutes for the first few days, then 10 minutes for the next few days. If things go well, you'll soon be reading for 30 minutes or even an hour.

Make sure to plan for temptation because it will arise. Program the remote for sleep mode at night. Then leave the remote in the kitchen so you don't succumb to the intoxicating blue light of the buttons when heading to bed. Social cognitive theory developed by Albert Bandura—a cornerstone of much of our understanding of how individuals interact with their environment—suggests that an individual's personal factors, such as expectations and goals, and environmental influences are equally reflected in their behavior[4]. Our environment is filled with triggers for old habits we want to change and lacks the triggers we need to reinforce our new habits. Make sure you place new cues throughout your living space to encourage your new habits, such as having enticing books on your bedside table.

Define and celebrate your actions, the changes you have made, and the mini-goals you have hit. Create specific goals based on what you learned from previous attempts. As you establish the habit, you can then add more small goals and celebration, minimizing the potential sabotage. Start a tracking system to celebrate each step of your newly-desired habits. Create consistency over intensity for a lifestyle of fitness success.

CHAPTER 3
THE REDEFIT MODEL

The RedeFit Model is what you've needed all along—a program based on you.

It's clear that the current health and fitness model is failing you. It sets up unrealistic expectations, leaving you exhausted and ashamed when you can't meet them. The model assumes your life is static and fails to adapt to its ever-changing nature. It shoves you into cookie cutter programs, ignoring your unique situation and goals. In taking such a narrow approach, it ignores the depth and breadth of your life. Enough already!

THE REDEFIT MODEL

You deserve so much better. And the good news is that you hold the answer in your hands. We call it the RedeFit Model. The name is derived from the notion of "**rede**fining **fit**ness." Yes, it's a bold statement, but well-justified. You'll soon understand why. The RedeFit Model is a major departure from what you're accustomed to and one that you'll finally be happy with. No longer will you be buried in a quagmire of information, in a place where your attention is so divided you can't make any headway.

Instead, the RedeFit Model will end your confusion and choice fatigue. You'll direct your time, energy, and focus in the direction of your goals. And you'll make real progress in real time. Say goodbye to unrealistic, unsustainable expectations heaped on you that only add to your burden. We know your days are full (that's an understatement) and you already wear many hats. You don't need *more* things to do. You just need the *right* things.

The RedeFit Model will clarify the areas that demand your focus—the ones that give you the best return on your investment of time and energy. It will be invigorating to focus on the essential aspects of your health and fitness.

Working on maintaining the right mindset will give you the best results and make the journey more enjoyable. A proper mindset can make the impossible seem possible.

You will no longer vainly attempt to fit your dynamic life into a static program. The RedeFit Model adjusts with you, allowing you to make steady progress toward your goals. As your life changes, the approach changes in response. How is this possible? Simple. The RedeFit Model is unlike anything you've seen. It's what you've needed all along—an approach based on you. It fits into your life and not the other way around.

The RedeFit Model has two parts:
1. An assessment
2. A customized path based on your assessment results

A path customized for you is one of the many things that sets the RedeFit Model apart. Unlike other models, you'll provide information on your goals, your current state, and your next step that will shape the approach for you. Other approaches expect you to fit into their mold. But we know **you need an approach based on you**. After all, you know yourself better than anyone else, so you should be the chief architect in building your success. The information you provide in the assessment will be instrumental in shaping the process and outcome of your unique journey.

TEN DISTINCT CATEGORIES

The RedeFit Model is comprised of ten distinct categories. A nice blend of all ten will help create the fitness outcomes and life balance you seek. When you take the assessment, you will evaluate yourself in these categories. You'll have the opportunity to gauge each category based on your goals and expectations. Knowing that you're in the driver's seat—that your true aims are the objective of the RedeFit Model—will be a refreshing experience. We'll provide you with all the foundational knowledge you need to gauge yourself in each category and steer your efforts in the direction of your goals.

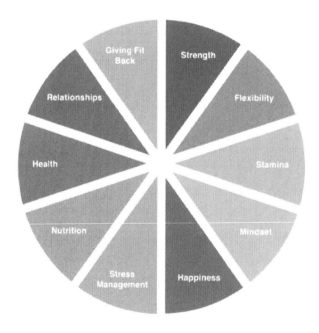

The ten categories are as follows:

1. Mindset
2. Stress Management
3. Happiness
4. Relationships
5. Nutrition
6. Health
7. Strength
8. Stamina
9. Flexibility
10. Giving Fit Back (GFB)

Ten different categories can seem a bit overwhelming at first glance, but don't worry. The RedeFit Model is meant to simplify your life. With a closer look at the ten categories, we can see that the ten categories represent two major components—physical and lifestyle. The physical component of the Redefit Model encompasses three categories: strength, stamina, and flexibility. The lifestyle component of the RedeFit Model includes nutrition, health, relationships, mindset, happiness, stress management, and giving fit back. We've designed this so you won't take on too much at once. Based on your assessment results, you'll place your focus on just one element from each facet—one physical and one lifestyle category. You can relax knowing that the results from your assessment answers are tailored to help you achieve your desired progress. As you progress and enter new seasons of your life, you can re-evaluate yourself and make the necessary course corrections. The RedeFit Model will meet your evolving goals and needs at each leg of your journey.

Most people have not been taught how to set goals. It's not as simple as stating our goals and then achieving them.

Once you've identified your top priority for physical and top priority for lifestyle, those will be your focus for the next four weeks. You might be unclear as to why you are starting with a given category when it doesn't appear to be your primary focus. For example: why would mindset be important if your goal was to lose weight? We have several categories in this book, like mindset, that serve as a foundation for overall fitness. Addressing nutrition from the start might help us lose weight more quickly but it can also lead to short-term results if the proper lifestyle foundation isn't set. Establishing a proper mindset can give us a better starting point to tackle difficult categories, like nutrition.

Another example is that you can be strong, but inflexible, which means your range of strength is compromised. For example, people who only bench press weights get very strong at bench pressing but tightness prevents them from easily reaching behind their bodies and you simply can't be strong in an area you can't access. The goal is to be strong through a full range of motion.

It's important to ask: why am I ultimately getting fit?

Adequate support is a major contributor to your success. To meet your goals, consider getting more involved with the fitness community—maybe joining a yoga class, doing an online video, or learning from a coach. Assets like these can make your push toward a healthier lifestyle easier. Remember your first time doing any kind of physical activity was probably a little awkward, but once you learned what to do, it became very natural. What we are doing here is creating habits. We already have daily habits—some positive, some negative. Over time the goal is to replace habits that are not serving us with new habits that do. If we do this systematically, one at a time, we increase the chance that long-term habits, as opposed to short-term fixes, are developed. We want to create this fitness journey as a part of your life, not something you have to do, or are shamed into doing, or worse, something you avoid altogether.

A CLOSER LOOK AT THE REDEFIT CATEGORIES

Next, we will take a closer look at each of the ten categories, so you will have a better understanding of what you're scoring yourself on when you take the assessment. These categories have been carefully cultivated to optimize your health and fitness outcomes.

Mindset - This piece must be in place to properly execute the other nine pieces. Our self-esteem, self-worth, and desire to keep working toward our fitness goals are based on our mindset. Working on maintaining the right mindset will give you the best results and make the journey more enjoyable. A proper mindset can make the impossible seem possible.

Stress Management - Once we can manage our stress, we have the capacity to take on more tasks and be more content. Stress can disturb your sleep, make you crave unhealthy food, and create unhealthy habits. Think of stress as burning up the fuel you need for your journey. The more you can control it, the more fuel you'll have to work out, make the right choices, and resist temptation.

Happiness - It's important to ask the question: why am I ultimately getting fit? The goal of this book is not to assist you in becoming a professional athlete or even to compete in a fitness competition; it was written to help you become lean, healthy, and happy. If happy isn't included in this trio, what's the point? It's rare for someone to say happiness is one of their fitness goals, but we would argue it's at the root of all goals. We want to lose weight to boost our confidence, become stronger to maintain our active lifestyle, and have enough energy to accomplish our goals, which will help us achieve greater happiness in our lives.

Relationships - Without a person or group of people with whom to share our experiences, the journey will be less than ideal. Humans evolved in groups and crave belonging. The key is having relationships that push you toward your fitness goals rather than turning you away. Nurturing the right relationships or creating new ones on your fitness journey not only makes it easier but also more enjoyable.

Nutrition - This category might be the most confusing and the most difficult to change. But it must be addressed. We will cut through the confusion and give you actionable guidelines, so you can derive the most benefit from the least amount of work. Remember that with nutrition, basics are key.

Health - Health is comprised of the things we must do each day to achieve our optimal long-term well-being. If we injure ourselves by overtraining, fail to fuel ourselves properly with quality food choices, or are in a mentally weakened state because we compare ourselves to the beautiful people on social media, we are not setting the stage for optimal health. Taking a look at health is ensuring we are optimizing our wellness for our lifelong journey.

Strength - Strength is one of the best indicators of longevity. We've noticed a trend working with clients as they age. If they lack strength, they often become dependent on other people. To continue to perform daily activities and remain independent, strength must be a part of the program.

Flexibility - You're only as strong as your functional range of motion. It's impossible to be strong through a range of motion you can't move through. You can be strong in a short range of motion but being flexible gives you the opportunity to be strong through a full range of motion. Therefore, getting strong isn't the right goal; getting strong in an optimal range of motion is what you're shooting for. This also helps you prevent injury from poor posture. For example, tight pectoral muscles will make your shoulders round forward straining your upper back muscles and placing your shoulder joint in an awkward position. This increases your chance of injury. Remember: a certain level of flexibility allows you to do more daily.

Stamina - The physical aspects culminate into your ability to perform your daily activities. If you are strong and flexible but can't tolerate much movement, you will be limited in what you can do. Stamina training will enable to you keep up with your kids, continue involvement in social athletic events, and allow you to enjoy activities, such as a long hike.

We are not referring to exercise as a way to burn calories. Instead, we are more concerned with the long-term and day-to-day benefits that each category provides. As we age, we would like to stay active, play with our kids, move without pain, and remain independent. A balance of strength, flexibility, and stamina is key.

Giving Fit Back - At first glance, this concept may be a bit confusing. It asks the question: are you being a positive fitness influencer? You may not consider yourself an influencer, but we all are. The way we communicate, the food we choose to eat, and our fitness routine or lack thereof influence the people around us. By going on this journey, you will be giving fit back by setting an example and being an inspiration to those around you. That's the most exciting part of the RedeFit Model. Think about yourself and your friends and family all being lean, healthy and happy. You can help make that happen!

Before we explain the assessment, we want to make sure you are starting with the right mindset. The current model of fitness which just focuses on your weight, body fat, strength or other singular markers will lead you down a frustrating path. Taking our path to wellness and fitness will look very different from the typical approach. You might recognize one or two elements, but our overall approach is a radical departure from the norm. The RedeFit Model is a well-rounded holistic approach that will leave you feeling lean, healthy, and happy. Tackling your health and fitness holistically and focusing on one to two areas at a time will lead you down the right path to achieving the fitness results you've been seeking. You will become the best version of yourself through our attainable and sustainable format.

HOW DOES THE ASSESSMENT WORK?

We've created a system to help you find balance, set appropriate goals, and find your optimal path. When you take the assessment, we recommend not overthinking it. And try not to compare yourself to those around you or to the things you see on social media. This is for you only.

To take the assessment, go to TheRedeFit.com.

As you discover your top two priorities, it's important to note you don't have to stop your current health and fitness routine. For example, you can stick with your yoga practice even if strength is your focus. Or you can keep lifting weights if flexibility is your focus. You will have two options: first, dedicate more time to your fitness or second, cut down on what you're currently doing to make more time for your new focus.

TWO OPTIONS

At this point, you've taken your assessment and you know your top two priorities. You have two options. After you have read *Notes from the Doc*, you can get started right away and jump to the two chapters that are most relevant to you. Alternatively, if you prefer to learn about each section, read each chapter sequentially and you will get the full benefits from learning about the ten categories. The choice is yours.

NOTES FROM THE DOC

COMMITTING TO THE GOAL-SETTING PROCESS

As you embark on this journey and the corresponding two priorities, it is essential that we continue the discussion we started in Chapter 2 on goal setting. Most people have not been taught how to set goals. It's a term frequently used by parents, teachers, coaches, and bosses as if it's a simple concept and one we should understand and be able to implement. Yet, goal setting is not as simple as stating our goals and then achieving them. And, if you think about it, we don't really need research to prove that. Conducting a survey 30 days after people make their New Year's resolutions would more than demonstrate that. When you look at the research in many fields like psychology, it shows that effective goal setting requires very specific behaviors. I introduced you to a few of these behaviors in my two previous *Notes from the Doc*. We will now take a closer look by exploring goal priming. Let's start by defining priming.

Priming

Priming in this context refers to a psychological term that represents key prompts and cues that are essential for learning and changing behavior [1]. Priming occurs in numerous ways impacting physical performance (i.e. personal trainers and coaches use it) as well as cognitive performance (i.e. educators and the media use it). In its basic form it represents creating associations that help in memory and action. For example, if you put a pen in your mouth horizontally this creates an expression associated with a smile [2]. Smiling has been shown to positively impact our emotions. In one study college students who read a comic strip with the pencil in their mouth found the strip significantly funnier on average than those with no pencil. Power posing—taking up more space—is highly associated with perception of dominance and power. Another common example is clothing. People can walk miles in basic cotton shorts with pockets. However, if you notice how people at your nearby trail or gym are dressed, they're wearing athletic wear. This isn't frivolous, but rather priming for behaviors outside the norm of daily routines and signaling the body to prepare for changes in heart rate, temperature, exertion, and challenge.

Throughout this book we will assist you in making new connections, strengthening existing connections, and even reframing a few. For example, when you think about changing your eating habits, are you thinking "diet" and in turn experiencing feelings of dread, sacrifice, and anticipating failure? To be successful with the RedeFit Model, we need to make sure those associations are sending your mind and body messages that support your goals. Let's move on to goal priming to break down the behaviors and corresponding messages I am referring to.

Goal Priming

Goal priming is the activation of a specific goal through situational cues. This, in turn, impacts how we process information around our goal and engage in behaviors toward that goal [3]. An example of situational cues are words we see in our environment. Have you noticed that many businesses have keywords or mantras that reflect the focus of that environment? Two examples are fitness centers and restaurants. When you enter gyms or workout facilities you often see motivational terms on the walls or pictures of people achieving goals. Restaurants frequently use decorations and pic-tures to denote the nationality of their food. For advertisers, this concept is essential to acquire the desired consumer behavior.

As I discussed in my notes in Chapter 2, mindfully establish-ing clear, specific, and challenging goals considerably increases the likelihood of success. Based on the well-established research and my many years of helping people achieve their goals, this is due to four primary reasons.

1. Goal-setting theory research shows that specific goals result in higher performance than setting no goals or even vague goals like "get more fit." *Specificity* in goal setting allows us to focus on ex-actly what we want to achieve through targeted activities at the moment and within a realistic timeframe. And just as important, it enables us to ignore activities that can rob us of focus and time. Furthermore, vague goals leave room for various interpretations as to whether the goal is attained. Our brains are wired to seek the path of least resistance. This increases the likelihood that we will interpret ourselves successful in some way, especially if it allows us to justify stopping something that is difficult.

2. The level of challenge associated with the goal corresponds to the level of individual performance. *Challenge* leads to an increase in effort and persistence to achieve the goal. It's important to be realistic about your ability. The challenge goal must truly be a challenge, but also take into account your personal resources. For example, an arthritic knee is an important consideration when set-ting a physical goal. In another example, one might want to eat 100 percent organic but live in a town with limited access to organic

foods or have a limited budget that does not support the higher food costs. On the flip side many people have had challenges achieving goals, especially those associated with fitness. This can set up unrealistic limitations in your mind regarding your abilities. When struggling to establish an appropriate level of challenge, seek out professionals that can provide individualized evaluation and trajectory as you meet your initial goals.

3. *Tracking progress* on goals is important. Accurate feedback on our progress keeps us from falling into traps of false perception. For example, if we are working on a nutrition goal but base our daily success on "feeling" like we did well because we don't think we had too much sugar increases the likelihood of encouraging behaviors not associated with our goal. Studies show that feedback regarding your results, making decisions based on your data, or competition with others have little impact on your behavior unless they lead to goal setting that is both specific and challenging. Being systematic in how you define your goals before you begin to track them is critical.

4. The combination of specificity, difficulty, and feedback is key to prompt us to find the best strategies to attain our goals. For example, if I want to reduce my stress, the specific goal is to find time to disengage from my stressors—the challenge being for at least ten minutes every day. Given these clear objectives, I can access *situational strategies* and environmental resources to accomplish this goal. So, although I might intend to set aside time before bed every day to de-stress, realistically I know that is not possible due to family routines or sheer exhaustion. I also realize that de-stressing

won't work during a commute with heavy traffic. However, getting up ten minutes earlier might work. Now, what can I do for ten minutes? Based on my personality and preferences, it might be a gratitude journal or meditation. Many diets, fitness routines, and de-stressors fail because we tend to adopt what has worked for someone else. But they are not us; they do not take into account our specific goals and resources. Situational strategies are successful when they are based on what is important to us, the resources we have, and our commitment based on the realistic feedback loop we have employed.

In each of the following chapters on the ten categories of RedeFit, we will provide specific information to help you recognize these cues and the behaviors that would support these areas. Accessing the key steps reviewed in this section will assist you in applying these behaviors and cues.

Chapter 4
Mindset

"Believe you can and you're halfway there.
–Theodore Roosevelt."

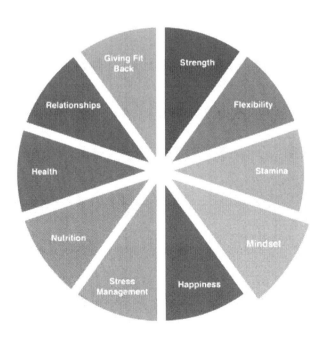

How you view the world, your life, and your fitness is solely based on your mindset. We all establish a set of attitudes towards the factors in our lives that determine how we choose to live. Mindset is influenced by where we grew up, our experiences, and the people around us, but it isn't carved in stone. We can actively participate in reshaping and refining it to better support our goals and efforts. Learning, traveling, meeting new people, and establishing new values are just a few ways to gain a new perspective and to change our mindset.

Why is mindset so important? The right mindset is the foundation for everything we want to accomplish. The right mindset is pivotal in initiating change. It is the key to getting started, to take the proverbial first step on the journey. The wrong mindset is an anchor that holds us back—keeping us stationary, unwilling to elicit change, and surrendering to inertia. The right mindset prompts us to consistently execute strategies moving us closer to our goals, whereas, with the wrong mindset, we constantly pull the reins in on positive change.

"Whether you think you can, or you think you can't, you're right." –Henry Ford

----

Here's an example that illustrates the importance of mindset. Below are quotes from two different clients on the same day and under the same circumstances.

"During the summer it's easier for me to eat healthy. There are more fresh fruits and vegetables. The weather is nice, so I'm more active, which makes me want to eat healthier."

"During the summer it's much harder for me to eat healthy. I like to enjoy a nice cold beer on a hot day. I have a friend with a pool, too, so there is typically drinking with lots of unhealthy snack options."

Contrasting comments like these are not unique. We often hear clients speak of life circumstances followed by a reason why it's better or why it's worse for their fitness goals—ideas conceived of by the person and their interpretation of their present conditions. These ideas eventually become their mindset. Take a moment to think about this for yourself: what is your mindset that detracts from your fitness goals? How do you approach your weekends, holidays, seasons of the year? What about sporting events? Do you tend to indulge more in unhealthy foods and exercise less when you're celebrating special occasions or socializing with friends?

Let's look at a daily ritual common to many. How do you treat yourself at the end of a hard work day? We've seen many people reward themselves with a drink or two every night. Other people go for a walk, take a bath, or read a book. The daily stressors we all share can be reduced with very different decompression strategies. The person drinking one to two drinks every night will be moving away from their fitness goals, whereas the person taking a walk every evening will be working toward their fitness goals—both accomplishing the task of winding down after a hard day. Your mindset determines your selection.

You are a direct reflection of the people you spend the most time with.

Show us your friends and we will understand your mindset. Your peer group reflects and influences your outlook, although it is ultimately up to you how you choose to think about things. And although you might spend time with people who have completely different mindsets than you, they also impact your outlook. Grandma was right when she said, "Birds of a feather flock together."

Take a moment to think about your closest friends and associates—your tribe. Reflect on the impact they have on you. Does their mindset positively or negatively influence your fitness goals? For example, do your friends urge you to try a new yoga class, or do they entice you to sample treats at a new pastry shop? Do they invite you to meet for coffee and talk about how great their new relationship is or to meet for cocktails and complain about work? We are social creatures whose mindset is influenced by those around us. Consider the people in your life and ask yourself: is this the right tribe for me? And, although you may be attached to your tribe, it might not serve your health and happiness goals.

"Many of our beliefs originate from how we were raised. Yes, it really does start with your family of origin. Your childhood shaped beliefs about yourself and what's possible."
–Notes from the Doc

MINDFULNESS BECOMES YOUR MINDSET

Your mindset is shaped by your past experiences. Therefore, to alter your mindset you must be present, intentional, and mindful. It has been said that 45 percent of waking behavior is habitual. Being mindful means not deferring to habit. Mindfulness is being consciously aware of what you are doing, which takes effort. It means asking yourself, *why am I doing this? Is this the best thing for me?* Being mindful makes you acutely aware of your surroundings and prompts you to look more deeply at what you are doing and why you are doing those things. This, in turn, creates new experiences, new perspectives, and helps adjust your mindset to one that is more positive and productive.

"Think about your past efforts that didn't work out. What have you learned from those about yourself and your lifestyle?" – **Notes from the Doc**

KNOWING YOURSELF

In nearly every chapter of this book we stress that knowing yourself, especially your personality tendencies, is critical in helping to define and determine the best lifestyle approaches for you. For example, if you are a people pleaser, you will feel inclined to make the people around you happy even at the expense of your wants and needs. This is not a bad quality but one to be aware of. You must be even more selective about the people you spend time with. So, for example, if you aim to please people who have unhealthy habits, such as smoking and partying, you will feel pressure to partake, even if it's detrimental to your health goals. Or perhaps you're the type of person who delights in being the center of attention, the life of the party—the person everyone wants to be around. You like to impress others, which often occurs by prompting people to do more of what they enjoy, such as having extra drinks during happy hour or running a couple more miles during a training run. Which one would you rather be a part of?

IT'S ALL RELATIVE

We live in a world of comparisons and benchmarks. Comparisons open our eyes to the incredible things people can accomplish. After all, a big part of success is belief in what's possible. Many people never try to reach their goals because the road seems too long and treacherous. Others fail to begin because the goal seems impossible. This is where comparison can be invaluable. If someone else has accomplished a goal, we know it is humanly possible. And, if it is humanly possible, it is within our grasp to accomplish the goal as well. Comparison shows us the potential for greatness and motivates us to try to achieve it.

But comparison is a double-edged sword. Comparisons can make us feel insignificant because we can always find someone with greater achievements. Think of a time you accomplished something, such as finishing a 5k run, losing 10 pounds, or attending a new fitness class. Then when basking in pride over your accomplishment, a colleague said they ran a 10k, lost 20 pounds or had been going to the same workout class for the past five years. How did this make you feel? The comparison doesn't diminish your success, but for many people it would make them feel less proud of their accomplishment. To use comparison effectively, it should be based on you—what you are trying to achieve and your improvements. Drawing inspiration and learning from others is great but judging their accomplishments relative to yours is not. Instead, maintaining a positive mindset and having little wins is critical to long-term success.

Benchmarks are standards from our past that we use as a measuring stick. In the fitness industry, one of the most popular benchmarks is some specific number on the scale, such as an individual's weight at high school graduation or on their wedding day.

"Our life is what our thoughts make it." –Marcus Aurelius

These are two very memorable moments and typically times during which our weight was the lowest in adulthood. Fast forward to today—20 birthdays, several jobs, and two children later. Perhaps you are now 20 pounds heavier. Can you lose that weight? Yes. Can you get in better shape than your 18-year-old self? Yes. Should you use your lighter weight as the benchmark for your goal weight? No. Why put that pressure on yourself? Setting your mind on the outcome instead of the process is a recipe for disaster. Again, staying positive and setting realistic expectations will help reinforce the right mindset and the right mindset will help you accomplish the right goals.

We can't emphasize enough the importance of the right mindset for the quality and productivity of your life. The right mindset helps you set appropriate goals, steers you in the right direction, and keeps you going when you're challenged. You must constantly check and reset your mindset. How? By being mindful of yourself and your body, environment, friends, and the little things you do every day. Being aware of those things will help you shape the right mindset for achieving your goals. This vigilance takes some effort, but it is a cornerstone for your success.

The table below presents recommendations for improving your mindset. In the ADD column, we propose behaviors to add to your daily activities. In the LIMIT column, we include behaviors to limit in your daily activities.

ADD
Find a few minutes each day to meditate.
List people, events, and things you're thankful for in a daily gratitude journal.
Recognize and celebrate small wins.
LIMIT
Limit activities that aren't serving you or helping you grow.
Avoid making excuses for yourself.
Pay attention to your internal dialogue and limit negative self-talk.

For a deeper understanding of these and other strategies, visit TheRedefit.com.

NOTES FROM THE DOC

A GROWTH MINDSET AND WHY WE WANT IT

Contrary to what some believe, the brain is not a muscle; it's an organ. The reason for this misconception is that much like muscles, the brain can be strengthened with use. When we consistently challenge our muscles, they strengthen and reach new limits. On a basic level, the same happens with your brain. Much like the endorphin high that occurs when people exercise their muscles, research indicates a strong correlation between the active, highly engaged use of the brain and happiness, specifically, the act of constantly learning, constantly mastering new and difficult tasks and persistence. [1] Psychologists call this a "growth mindset."

Mindset research divides people into two primary groups: those with a fixed mindset and those with a growth mindset. Those with a fixed mindset believe that character, creativity, performance, and intelligence are static. They tend to assume their level of intelligence is fixed—that they either understand or know a given level of information, and other people have more or less. Understandably, most of us have been taught that IQ is a fixed number that does not change. While as you mature your score on standardized IQ tests may not appreciatively evolve, that does not mean your overall intelligence does not. Furthermore, when we believe our intelligence is fixed, this perception functionally erodes our motivation to learn and to be engaged. This is further exacerbated by societal tendencies to praise the ability and not the effort. So, when praise comes in the form of ability, (you're so smart) as opposed to effort (your persistence to solve problems is amazing), we tend to give up more quickly when we do not instantly understand something. People with a fixed mindset are often more oriented to external things, plans, and people to achieve their fitness goals. The underlying assumption is that they cannot grow as an individual and the answer lies outside themselves.

Now ask yourself the following question: who is more valuable on a team? Is it someone who is considered smart but won't engage when things get hard? Or is it someone who works hard and persists until the problem is solved? Of course, it's the persistent one with a growth mindset. They believe that habits and characteristics are not static; rather they are flexible and can be worked on. They tend to focus on small gains, longer systematic processes, and increased success over time. They do not view failures as setbacks; instead, they view them as growth opportunities. They approach critiques as learning experiences, and they view effort as the key to mastery. They understand that we can continue to develop through practice, dedication, and effective mentoring. These people are highly engaged in learning, especially in light of adversity—and remain happy.

So, what is your mindset about getting fit? What is the mindset of those around you? Do you assume that once you are a parent, or over 40, your body and health will go downhill? Do you view aging as a fixed state? Or do you believe in redefining aging, learning more about your maturing body, and identifying ways to optimize it at each life phase? Are you limiting yourself based on expectations of others (i.e. pretty girls don't lift weights) or are you a sponge soaking up as much information you can to tailor your efforts? The fact that you're reading this book indicates that if you don't already have a growth mindset, you are off to a good start. Think about your past efforts that didn't work out. What have you learned from those about yourself and your body and lifestyle? Did you remember to praise yourself for your past and current effort, or is your mindset fixed? I cannot do this. I am not disciplined. I am not...

"For twenty years my research has shown that the view you adopt for yourself profoundly affects the way you lead your life. It can determine whether you become the person you want to be and whether you accomplish the things you value."
–Carol Dweck

So, how do we attain and keep a growth mindset? Leading researchers have linked this to the beliefs we have about ourselves or the story we tell ourselves.

We have all tried to adopt a new perspective. Why is it so hard? Many of our beliefs originate from how we were raised. Yes, it really does start with your family of origin. Your childhood shaped beliefs about yourself and what's possible. The ones that hold you back need some rewiring. Scientists in the areas of neurology and psychology have shown we can change our beliefs and build new neural pathways in our brain to strengthen and expand our new beliefs. There are several ways to do this. For our purposes here, I am going to focus on two–your environment and your language.

In other chapters we talk about evaluating your tribe—those you spend time with as part of your fitness journey to reach and maintain your goals. Research indicates that because mindset can be changed, the behavior of a tribe can evolve when the leader of the tribe adjusts their mindset and the environment changes. This is critical because sometimes you can't change who is in your tribe, nor do you want to, such as when it's your family. As a result, impacting your tribe is the best way to move toward your fitness goals and support loved ones.

For example, let's say you are the primary cook in your family or leader of the tribe in food-related matters and you often eat in front of the television. You can change what you cook and where you eat to support healthier habits of the tribe. Perhaps in your circle of friends you tend to follow suggestions instead of making them. You value your friendships, but the suggested places and activities are not consistent with your fitness goals. How might you lead more with suggestions of healthier and more active places? Remember, change is a process and you are building new neural pathways, so approach it in stages. For example, you want to do yoga, and your friends want to catch up over a beer. Find a yoga class at a brewery. Drink less, do more. Over time, you can go to yoga together and then enjoy a healthy smoothie or coffee instead. Help your friends modify their mindsets to one of growth to explore more and redefine the tribe's fitness.

To impact our personal beliefs and environments, we must pay close attention to both internal and external language. Our self-talk impacts our perceptions, mindset, and outcomes. Do we really hate something, or is it just a difficult challenge that requires finding a way to break the task down into more manageable steps toward mastery? Are we failing at dieting, or have we not found a nutrition and lifestyle plan that works for us? Do we suck at running, or have we never been trained to run for our body type and stamina levels? Do we have no willpower, or do we just need support in creating environments and opportunities to reduce temptations? If we took our car to the mechanic and they indicated they weren't going to fix it because it was a piece of junk, would we accept that and not drive our car? Of course not. We would likely go to another mechanic with a growth mindset who would problem-solve until finding a solution. We must treat ourselves the same way. It's best to view our setbacks as efforts toward learning more about ourselves and our needs. We need to communicate with others and ourselves that which would make us stronger and better. We must embrace that there is so much to learn, experience, and achieve if we put our mind to it!

CHAPTER 5
STRESS MANAGEMENT

"The more we fill our bucket with gratitude, the less likely we are to stay sensitized to stress and send the fight-flight signal to our body." –Notes from the Doc

----

When reading the title of this chapter, you may have nodded knowingly and heaved a deep sigh. Stress. The word alone might make you feel tense. It may evoke images of a frantic and chaotic mind attempting to tackle fifteen things at once. Stress leaves you frustrated, exhausted, and anxious. We've all been there. And because of that, we would like a stress-free life. Right?

Not so fast. A moderate amount of stress is actually necessary for life. It's even a requirement in achieving many of our goals. Working out stresses the body, gravity stresses our bones, and learning new activities can beneficially stress our mind helping us to live a healthier and happier life.

The key is not to eliminate stress but to learn how to manage it. To do so we need to truly understand it. We classify stress into three main categories: negative, positive, and perceived. There are also five different origins of stress that we face in our lives: personal, work, sleep, nutrition, and exercise.

NEGATIVE STRESSORS

To most of us, the term "negative stress" probably sounds redundant. This is our default notion when we refer to stress. There are indeed some stressors that are purely negative. A serious injury, physical or mental abuse, losing a loved one, or many of the unforeseen problems that change the path we are on. Thankfully, we can make the best out of most situations and seek help and guidance when needed.

"We can choose how we perceive a situation, even when there are clear negatives. We have a choice about how much of our mental energy for how long we spend on the negative vs. the potential positives." –Notes from the Doc

----

Interestingly, one common denominator shared by many inspirational and successful people is that they have had significant setbacks in their lives. They experienced significant negative stressors and overcame them, propelling them to even greater heights. There are countless stories of extremely successful people that came from nothing, had major setbacks, or dealt with life-changing trauma. Oprah Winfrey was born into poverty in rural Mississippi. Celine Dion was the youngest of 14 children in a low-income family. Demi Moore was raised by her alcoholic mother and stepfather. Steve Jobs was fired by his own company. Walt Disney was told that no one would ever like Mickey Mouse. But we know these people not only survived their hardships and woes; they went on to become wildly successful. The common assumption is that all negative stressors will have a long-lasting negative effect, but it doesn't have to be that way. The truth is: it depends upon what we do with it.

POSITIVE STRESSORS

Positive stressors may be a novel notion to you. "Positive" and "stress" don't belong together—right? It seems like a contradiction of terms. However, there are many positive stressors that contribute to our well-being. We include three examples of positive stressors for the body on the RedeFit Model—strength, stamina, and flexibility. If overdone or performed improperly, they can become negative stressors. Assuming you are following our plan or a beneficial training program, we will keep strength, stamina, and flexibility in this "positive stressors" category. For muscles and bones to become stronger some stress must be applied. Think of astronauts in outer space. The lack of gravity, which normally creates resistance or stress on the body, triggers bone and muscle loss for them. As in the case of gravity's effect on the body, stress is needed to strengthen many things.

Just like in the physical realm, there can be positive mental stressors as well. Think about the last time you traveled to a new place or learned something new. Both experiences can be stressful because of the unknown and the effort of acquiring new knowledge or skills. When you learn new activities, you grow as an individual, become more comfortable with new situations, and you stretch yourself. Each time it becomes a little easier.

It is important to remember that there will be some discomfort with positive stressors as with negative stressors. In other words, positive stressors are not necessarily a walk in the park; there's no escaping some level of hardship. What distinguishes negative and positive stressors is the result. If the discomfort brought about some benefit or growth, it was a positive stressor.

PERCEIVED STRESSORS

This is the most important stress category. As with so many things in life, whether you think something is a stressor or not, you are correct. It's all about your perception. We can turn almost every event, every day, every moment into a positive or negative stressor. Yes, there are truly negative stressors that can't be perceived any other way, which we will discuss later in this chapter. But, for the most part, we have control over how we respond to events or situations.

Think about the things you may consider stressors in your life, such as a traffic delay on your morning commute to work. When you see brake lights and slowing traffic, you may start to feel anxious, frustrated, or upset. What if, instead, being stuck in traffic signaled a moment to enjoy your favorite song, relish solitude, or listen to your favorite audiobook?

Next, think about the last time you had an argument with someone close to you. You may have felt annoyed or misunderstood. But what if you had seen it as an opportunity to learn something new about your loved one, take in a new perspective, or practice patience and love? Focusing on negative stress could weaken your relationship but practicing patience and love could strengthen your bond. That is the gift of stress. When approached properly, it can spur growth. What makes it even more powerful is how you use it, which is your choice.

Having explored the ideas of negative stress, positive stress, and perceived stress, it's clear that the topic of stress is not all about negative stress. Contrary to what so many believe, we don't want to eliminate stress from our lives. Rather, we want to manage it. Some stress is needed for us to live and even required to achieve many of our goals. A requisite to managing stress is understanding it, so let's explore the origins.

FIVE ORIGINS OF STRESS

The five origins are: personal, work, sleep, nutrition, and exercise. Classifying stressors into five origins allows us to more easily examine different areas of our life. By doing this, we can identify the areas that are lacking and the ones creating the most negative stress. After exploring the five origins of stress, you will have another tool for creating significant and lasting change.

Personal

Our personal lives are filled with situations that can mitigate or increase stress. Getting married, having a good friend, and enjoying hobbies, or getting divorced, overworking and not having any fun are just a few examples of each. How much stress we experience with each event depends on our perception of the event. Getting married can be one of the best days of your life or one of the most stressful. If you're worried about pulling off a perfect day, pleasing your guests, and not spending more than your budget allows, your wedding could be very stress-inducing. If you approach the event with clear and realistic expectations, it could be a memory you cherish forever.

Because the human brain has evolved with a tribe-like mentality, your sense of belonging is extremely important. Your inclusion and standing in the tribe can enhance your happiness and decrease your level of stress. Your happiness isn't necessarily reliant on your status within the tribe as much as inclusion in the group. The tribe offers a sense of shared experience and fellowship. One of the best ways to create and grow a sense of belonging is giving back, whether it's helping at a homeless shelter, an after-school children's program, or a soup kitchen. Helping others, being with people you trust and can be yourself with, and working toward a common goal fosters a sense of belonging. This can be with your sports team, at your fitness club, a charity you volunteer with, or on the job. The extent of group activity that's comfortable will depend on your personality—introverted vs. extroverted—but even the most introverted people share DNA that's encoded with tribe-based survival instincts.

Another way to mitigate stress is to set aside time to have fun. Not building fun into your life can be a real problem. All too often our calendars are filled with obligations with no time for fun or restoration. Planning fun is one of our top recommendations for helping people manage their stress. We encourage you to schedule fun time in your calendar. If you are not used to planning fun, this can be difficult at first.

"Rank order your list of things you would enjoy doing based on desires, preference, and cost. Plug these into your life accordingly. Joy comes in all sizes."—Notes from the Doc

----

Planning for fun offers two distinct advantages. First, scheduling fun time gives you the opportunity to eagerly anticipate the future and the enjoyable activities that await you. Second, you get to engage in activities that enrich your life. Think back to when you were a child. What were some things you enjoyed? Did you play an instrument, go to a vacation cabin, or play cards? What would you like to do again? Before you had a full-time job and children, what did you do for fun? Did you go on boat rides, hike, or go out dancing? What would you like to do again? What is something new you would like to do? Do you have a special place you'd like to visit? Once you've decided what would add fun to your life, start planning right away!

Increasing your fun quotient is essential. There will be negative stressors no matter how positive you are, but if you balance those events with plenty of me-time—time alone doing what you love, and we-time—time with people close to you doing what everyone enjoys—then you will live a healthier and happier life with well-managed stress.

Work

"For there is nothing either good or bad but thinking makes it so."
–William Shakespeare.

As we all know, our professional lives can be a hotbed for stress. It represents our very livelihood and at least a third of every week-day. It can include situations such as getting a new job, receiving a promotion, acquiring a new client, losing a client, or getting laid off. As with our personal lives, much of your stress response to a work situation will be predicated on your perception of the event. A new job could give you financial independence and a purpose. Conversely, a new job could mean doing something you don't en-joy doing or working with people you don't care for.

Work is like the other origins of stressors in our lives. It can bring truly negative stressors into your life, such as an abusive boss or bullying coworkers. When situations like these arise, carefully assess them and decide if it's time to move on. More often, though, work stressors are reminiscent of Shakespeare's line, "For there is nothing either good or bad, but thinking makes it so." Many

situations and conditions that arise at work aren't easily catego-
rized as positive or negative. There is fluidity in their classifica-
tion based on our perceptions. For example, a tight deadline on a
project isn't decidedly positive or negative. It might function as a
negative stressor, disrupting your sleep, causing your mind to race,
and elevating your heart rate. The same tight deadline can also be
a positive stressor that hones your focus, helps you discover new
capacities, and is a catalyst for growth. It can challenge you to do
more than you thought possible and grow from the experience.

----

*Remember, even positive stressors include some level of
discomfort, so see those positive stressors through to the end.
You're sure to be rewarded.*

Steering work stressors toward the positive end of the spectrum
require a moment of self-reflection. We often forget how much
effort went into attaining our current professional position. We
worked hard to overcome obstacles and to meet the many obligations on our calendars. It's helpful to remember that many people,
and even the younger you, would be happy to have the work stressors that currently await you.

Another way to reframe work stressors is to take a moment
to ask yourself if the situation or condition you're currently con-
fronted with allows you to grow and learn. Often you will find
the answer is "yes." In that case, it shouldn't be avoided, but embraced. This is an opportunity for you to grow, to expand your
skill set, and to showcase your amazingness. And, remember,

even positive stressors include some level of discomfort, so see those positive stressors through to the end. You're sure to be rewarded.

Sleep

Sleep, a cornerstone of health and well-being, is often overlooked. A good night's sleep is one of the best ways to manage stress throughout the day. After a rough night of sleep, we're irritable, we have a short temper, and we're generally less pleasant to be around. We've all been there. A lack of quality sleep can negatively affect hormonal and neurotransmitter production. This results in less energy, less focus, improper food regulation, and a whole host of other issues that stress the body.

There is some good news about sleep. Thankfully, sleep is something many of us have control over. Sleep hygiene, sleep routine, food and supplementation, and hours of sleep are just a few factors that can majorly affect sleep quality, many of which you can influence.

Sleep hygiene starts with setting up your bedroom for sleeping success. Aim to make your bedroom a dark, distraction-free, comfortable environment that supports restorative sleep. Simple— right? Hang curtains to block outside light, keep the bedroom TV-free (at least before bedtime), and set the temperature to a setting you find pleasant to sleep. With the ambiance established, your pre-bed routine requires examination.

A good sleep routine consists of a two-part approach to prepare you for some restorative sleep. The first part of a well-constructed sleep routine is a nightly regimen that helps you calm down from the day and prepares your body for sleep. This may include such things as a few minutes of meditation, a gratitude journal, an evening walk in the setting sun, or simply deep breathing. Since the goal is to wind down, the second part of a smart sleep routine is avoiding things that are stimulatory. This includes such simple interventions as avoiding screen time before bed (the light makes your brain thinks it's day and time to be awake) and limiting caffeine intake. Find practices that help you wind down and avoid anything stimulatory.

This a good place to note evening food and supplementation. In general, avoid foods that cause stomach rumbling or an upset stomach. Some common culprits are dairy and spicy foods. An angry tummy is a surefire way to inhibit falling and staying asleep. If you've got all the other ducks in a row and you're still struggling to get restorative sleep, it might also be time to explore supplementation. Many people benefit from magnesium or melatonin to help them wind down, drift off to sleep, and stay asleep until the rooster crows.

One final important aspect of controlling sleep is giving yourself the opportunity to get the right amount of sleep. Setting up your schedule to get the recommended seven to nine hours of sleep isn't always realistic. With the many obligations we juggle, we may have to make tradeoffs like leaving the dirty dishes for the next day or saving your unread emails for the morning. But seven hours may be an unattainable goal at this point in your life. Nevertheless, try the strategies presented here to maximize your sleep.

Nutrition

Nutrition can be a powerful tool for managing stress and aiding recovery. It can also be a catalyst for diminishing health and increased stress. Eating too much or too little food stresses the body. Inadequate nutrient intake and not eating enough protein or fat is stressful on the body. In our chapter on nutrition, we detail how to eat for optimal health, but here are the main points to remember. Drink plenty of water, eat lots of vegetables, get adequate fat and protein, and don't overeat. Details about the optimal food quantity are featured in our chapter on nutrition. Our most important recommendation: eat real food. We could have amazing relationships, good quality sleep, and love our work, but if we don't eat right, we could be stressing our bodies unnecessarily. Fortunately, it is one aspect of our health we can fully control.

Exercise

Exercise is a stressor, particularly strength and endurance training. This stressor can be hugely impactful for our well-being. It can strengthen our bones, help us build muscle, and enable us to perform our daily tasks with ease. When it comes to exercise, you must be careful about doing too much, especially when starting a new workout routine. This goes back to a major theme throughout this book—consistency over intensity. Be conservative in your approach to exercise.

How much exercise you can handle depends greatly on how well you manage your other stressors. It depends greatly on the quality of your nourishment and sleep, your current workout routine, and the stress levels in other areas of your life. The more on point these other factors are, the more you can work out without leading to injury or burnout. For example, if you had a poor night's sleep, didn't eat the most nutritious food, and you're on a stressful work deadline, then maybe swapping your demanding exercise routine for a stretch, a light run, or a long walk would be best. On the other hand, if you had a good night's sleep, were able to eat properly, and the other major stressors are in check, then you can tackle a long, hard workout that might include strength and stamina exercises.

Our big takeaway from this chapter is not all stress is bad and it is largely dependent on your perception. Bad stressors can turn out better than we had thought. In reality, you only have control over what you are going to do next. In our recommendations on how to improve your stress management, we will be adding more fun activities to your life, more sleep, daily physical activity, and more reflection to slow down and think through what's going on.

"Research shows that taking even a few minutes and stepping away from what is overwhelming is essential to reducing your stress response and gives you the space you need to put the trigger in perspective." –Notes from the Doc

----

The table below presents recommendations for managing stress. In the ADD column, we propose behaviors to add to your daily activities. In the LIMIT column, we include behaviors to limit in your daily activities.

ADD
Increase the amount of sleep you get each night.
Designate more "me-time"/decompression time.
Enjoy more quality/"we-time" opportunities.

LIMIT
Avoid using electronics 30 minutes before bed.
Minimize complaining and negative language.
Be mindful of how often and to whom you say yes.

For a deeper understanding of these and other strategies, visit TheRedefit.com.

NOTES FROM THE DOC

In a 2014 Harris poll on behalf of the American Psychological Association of over 3000 Americans, 78 percent of people say they have experienced at least one health symptom of stress, and over a third experienced sadness or depression within the last month as a result. Additionally, more individuals than in previous years reported being in poor health [1]. We know that our brain is built to engage stress responses when we feel imminent danger; this is by design to trigger our bodies into the fight-flight mode for a short-term burst, so we can effectively and acutely react. However, when we engage in this mode over long periods of time, due to intense stress, we negatively impact our bodies and mind. Knowledge is power and it's important to learn how to avoid and respond to this tendency. As such, a significant focus of this chapter has been on the types of stress and how we perceive it. This is because we have much more control and capacity to deal with stress than most of us believe. We have the ability to define and interpret our stress. So, for instance, meditation might reduce one person's stress but perhaps not yours. Is it because you cannot meditate? No, you can definitely learn to meditate. It may have more to do with the type of stress and your mindset.

As I write this piece on stress, I am just beginning my annual family vacation. And I am stressed—how will I finish this piece? I know I am stressed because I broke out in hives, my stomach is upset, my breathing is shallow, and I am sporting a nagging headache. So, your first thought might be, well, of course, you're not supposed to work on vacation. You're just adding to your stress. Typically, I would agree. However, in reviewing the types and origins of stress we've discussed in this chapter, I have quickly come to realize that my work deadline is not the sole contributor to my current state of mind.

I am also thinking about food I might have eaten that contributed to my symptoms or noting that traveling takes a toll. I realized that I alone created my stress. I love our annual trip—the location, being near people I care deeply about, and the opportunity to breathe and reflect. However, I am a people pleaser. I want to make sure everyone has a good time and is happy. With that goal in mind, I worried about the potential for rain in the forecast, racked my brain to make sure I had the right food and activities, discouraged because some family members decided not to come, and wondered if I may have rented a vacation home not everyone will like. And, of course, I have some work deadlines. All these worries stirring in my mind are making my body sick.

It would be amazing if I could gain perspective and see myself doing this. I have been at this stress game for a long time, and you would think I'd catch myself. Sometimes I do. But often I don't and then I must play catch up. Furthermore, I am told to "stop stressing out" and "stop worrying." Easier said than done—right? The reality is that my strength is people, reading them and responding to their needs. It fuels me, and I do not want to change, but that does not mean I am powerless to mediate the challenges that accompany my strength. We all have our strengths and they vary amongst us. People who are natural leaders, problem solvers, worker bees, the life of the party, or the calm and steady types can all experience stress resulting from their strengths being over-taxed. There are many research-based strategies for coping with these over-extensions of ourselves. The following are three I used to get me back on track for this vacation—ones that I often recommend to my clients.

PERSPECTIVE

I recently overheard an older gentleman saying to a teenage boy, "Just you wait, child, you don't know what stress is." Most "mature" adults often look back at their early adulthood years fondly—reminiscing about the more carefree season of their life. Why is that? Is it because it is easy being a teenager or a young adult? Is there no stress in learning how to drive, trying to have control over your life when you don't, learning how to date and develop real friendships, taking out student loans, or working for minimum wage? We know the answer is: no, of course not. Or there would not be widespread teen depression, bullying, or worse, suicide—to name a few of the modern-day challenges facing our youth. Then why does it seem we feel more stressed than ever as we age?

The answer is in large part linked to our perceptions. Stress is not only cumulative, but it functions like an allergy. As people develop allergies, it takes much less exposure to allergens, such as cat hair, pollen, and nuts, to create the same allergic response. Over time the allergic response can get even worse given the same level of exposure. Stress functions in the same way. Research has shown that exposure to stress over time rewires the brain, leaving it less agile to respond to new situations, keeping it in a constant state of anxiety or even triggering mood disorders [2]. So, for example, eventually our body's stress response to the daily commute traffic jam is the same as its response to a life-or-death situation. Imagine the level of stress response on the body every time you are running late, someone says something negative, or you miss a deadline at work!

To combat this, we need to be proactive in the messages we send to our body. Let's reflect on my current situation. As I mentioned before,

I have had ample years to fine-tune my ability to be stressed; I have been sensitized to this allergic reaction and my body responded quickly. Because of that, I got worked up way too quickly and easily. I did not stop and think about my vacation circumstances before diving right into it, rather, I sent my body the signal to respond to catastrophic stress. I need to acknowledge that everyone in my family expressed excitement when I showed them the house we were renting online. For those that couldn't come, I should note that they appreciated being included. Also, I need to acknowledge how fortunate I am to be able to include everyone. For those that did come, even if they had a great experience only 50 percent of the time, that was still significantly more time than I would have spent with them had we not gone on vacation. We can choose how we perceive a situation, even when there are clear negatives. We have a choice about how much of mental our energy for how long we spend on the negative vs. the potential positives.

MAKE A PLAN

Stress becomes a problem when the demands placed on us exceed our ability to process and execute. So, when the day has been long, and the children will not go to sleep, cleaning up after dinner can wait. You technically could clean it up at that moment. But if you are mentally or physically drained, your greatest accomplishment in that moment should be simply not taxing yourself further. It is nice to wake up to a clean kitchen, but if your body is in overdrive stress mode, you will not sleep well, and you won't wake up feeling refreshed, regardless of what greets you. Research shows that taking even just a few minutes and stepping away from what is overwhelming is essential to reducing your stress response and gives you the space needed to put the trigger into perspective. Then, before you reengage with your challenges, it is recommended that you make a plan [3].

A recent study of 3000 people across 30 countries including the United States indicated that the most successful strategy for managing stress was through planning [3]. This is because when we plan, including creating lists, timelines, and priorities, it allows us to foresee many things we miss in the moment. When we plan, we notice that our schedules are already full, we can better see how long some tasks will take, and it allows us to prioritize and not become overwhelmed. This planning helps us say "no" to taking on too much, or perhaps most importantly, "no" to those requests that are not consistent with what we value most. For example, a family may decide they want to be highly involved in their children's school to connect with their children in a meaningful way. However, if they are not planful, they may find that they are spending more time at school functions or tasks than actually spending quality time with their children. If your joy at work is contributing meaningfully to important projects, saying "yes" to every request of help from your coworkers may make your work suffer, further adding to your stress.

For some of us planning comes naturally. For others, it just causes more stress. As with anything in life, go for consistency over intensity and moderation. If you're planning your workday or preparing for a big transition, start where you can and try different tools to assist you. For example, I like lists. I spend a lot of time on my computer, so you would think I would make electronic lists, but I don't. I prefer to make lists on paper. I like to cross off items when they are complete and throw the paper away. It's not always efficient; sometimes I leave my list at home or at work or lose it. But overall, it's the best method for me.

Let's take a moment to revisit my vacation. I didn't want to plan out my days on vacation or make checklists of amazing moments I hoped to have. However, I needed to make a plan for the week before my vacation. Instead, I worked furiously to get everything done for work and the household. I said yes to everyone who wanted something since I would be gone for a week. As I packed at the last minute, I had a nagging feeling I did not get it all done. I left for vacation tired, stressed and overwhelmed, fantasizing that I would miraculously be calm and relaxed when I arrived.

GRATITUDE

Cicero defined gratitude as the "parent of virtues." Its presence in our lives enables us to cultivate more virtuous attitudes and behaviors. Gratitude is about marveling in what is instead of wishing for something different. It is often considered a personality trait—a state of being. Most of us who have access to this book or the RedeFit Model have so much to be grateful for. Our standard of living relative to many parts of the world is unmatched. Ironically, this can create a unique dilemma for those of us in the modern world. We are bombarded with media reminders of what others have and with external definitions of success. This media onslaught can trigger feelings of inadequacy and deprivation; we yearn for what others have and think attaining those things is the answer to our problems.

Gratitude is not the same as appreciation, indebtedness, or being thankful for the good things in life. Its essence is in marveling at what exists regardless of the bumps in the road; it's an appreciation for what life has to offer. The positive emotions that coexist with gratitude like empathy, joy, and calm serve to absorb our energies, stifling emotions like regret, sadness, and anxiety. Gratitude sets the standard for how we choose to fill our emotional and physical buckets.

Few will contest that a gratitude mentality is a good thing, but on some days it's easier to acknowledge it. However, whereas stress may work like an allergy, gratitude is your happy, healthy virus. It's contagious. Surrounding yourself with people, places, and daily reminders that reflect gratitude helps spread this amazing virus. We need frequent reminders to pause and express gratitude. It does not have to be time-consuming or be public, but it should be genuine. The more we fill our bucket with gratitude, the less likely we are to stay sensitized to stress and send the fight-flight signal to our body when we lose our car keys or have to pitch in at work due to a colleague's oversight.

When I cultivated a gratitude mentality, it did not take me long to recalibrate my vacation stress, marveling at what life had to offer and acknowledging the amazing people and opportunities in my life. This includes the incredible opportunity to contribute to others' wellness through this book.

CHAPTER 6
HAPPINESS

Happiness is approaching each moment with a sense of gratitude and serenity, allowing you to pursue your dreams and goals without risking your sense of well-being if they don't pan out.

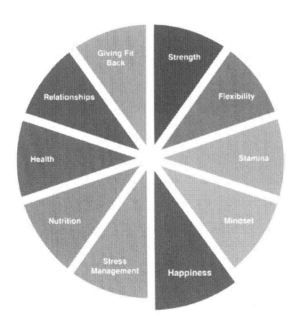

You may be asking, why is a happiness chapter in a fitness book? The simple answer lies in examining the comments we hear daily: "I want to lose weight." "If only I were stronger." "I'd like to be more toned." "I wish I were healthier." "I'd like to be more flexible." When we look more deeply at these comments, we know that what people really seek is happiness.

So, what is happiness and how do we determine what that looks like for each one of us? In this chapter, we want to help you answer these questions and in turn, make sure that an accurate definition of happiness for you helps determine what is realistic for your fitness goals.

DEFINING HAPPINESS

Let's start by defining happiness. It isn't as easy as it may seem because of the discrepancy between what people think it should be and what it actually is. There are several misconceptions. First, the media and popular culture portray happiness as intense moments of joy. While happiness can include moments of joy, these moments are peaks, such as graduating from college, landing our first job, getting married, having a child, or receiving a big promotion. Peak moments bring pleasure and elation into our life. But using peak moments as a measuring stick for happiness is flawed. Why? Peak moments aren't sustainable and don't happen consistently. And honestly, you wouldn't want them to. Can you imagine starting a new exciting job every week or welcoming a new baby into your family every month? Those moments of joy would be overwhelming, and you'd experience peak moment fatigue.

The infrequency of peak moments makes them special but also makes them a poor metric for defining happiness. If we measure happiness that way, we rarely feel happy. Using peak moments as our measuring stick sets up false expectations for our everyday life. By focusing on false expectations, you feel like you are falling short instead of enjoying the simple pleasures of daily living. Fortunately, happiness isn't limited to peak experiences.

Advertisers would have you believe that happiness lies in polishing off a container of your favorite ice cream, slipping on a new pair of jeans, or watching your favorite show. These experiences provide fleeting moments of gratification but fall short of true happiness. We believe happiness can last beyond the melting point of ice cream. Happiness can be enduring.

And lastly, there is the fairytale misconception of happiness. This idea holds that happiness is outside our control, that lucky individuals born under the right star and living in the just-right confluence of circumstances get to live happily ever after. The rest of us are out of luck. We all know people who seem to be the lucky recipients of happiness. It's easy to blame fate for others' happiness and our own unhappiness.

Yet, we know fairytales don't exist and those seemingly fortunate people are dealing with their own problems and obstacles even if it isn't obvious to us. The destructive part of this thinking is that it neglects the control we have over our emotional lives. And, although happiness can happen accidentally, we have far more control than we think.

The RedeFit Model helps redefine your pursuit of happiness. True happiness diverges from the aforementioned misconceptions and is signified by contentment. This does not mean settling or stagnating, nor does it mean giving up or lowering your standards. Instead, it is more appropriately defined as approaching each moment with a sense of gratitude and serenity, allowing you to pursue dreams and goals without risking your sense of well-being if they don't pan out. We all know that some things despite our best efforts just don't work out. And that should be okay. Without the pressure of perfection or the expectation of constant peaks, you are free to experience a lasting and pervasive sense of happiness. We will have peaks and valleys in our lives, but ultimately, we are looking for a life of contentment.

So, how do we achieve and sustain happiness? What must we avoid and what should we indulge? Let's examine some stumbling blocks on the road to happiness and then explore ways to cultivate happiness.

"Comparison is the thief of joy." –Theodore Roosevelt

There are activities and behaviors that can diminish happiness. Comparison is a big one. Too often we measure ourselves against others. Our thoughts may sound something like this:

"My best friend has a new car and mine is 10 years old."

"My cousin makes $30,000 more than I do."

"She can eat an entire cake without gaining a pound, and I gain five pounds by just looking at a piece."

And the list goes on. Rarely do these comparisons lead to a sense of happiness and fulfillment.

Comparison is further magnified by social media. We live in a world in which we constantly view the highlight reels of friends and acquaintances. Doesn't it seem like every time you access social media everyone is having the time of their lives—posting pics from their vacations, enjoying amazing relationships, raising perfect children, and celebrating having just landed their dream job? Meanwhile, we may be experiencing none of those things and wonder where things went wrong.

We may use our beautiful mind—capable of bringing immense positivity into the world—to seed discontent and unhappiness.

When we compare our accomplishments to others' apparent successes, we boost negative emotions about ourselves and others. We beat ourselves up for not having achieved their successes and resent them for having what we want. We feel bad about ourselves because we perceive that everyone else is doing better. We may use our beautiful mind—capable of bringing immense positivity into the world—to seed discontent and unhappiness.

Keep in mind that people tend to post their successes and achievements on social media, not their low points. As we've discussed, peak experiences alone don't make people happy. They occur too infrequently to bring enduring happiness. Instead, it's the response to everyday life that helps us to cultivate happiness. The good news is that comparison can be used to our advantage, which we'll explore later in this chapter.

There is no such thing as doing it all, and by trying, we are mentally imploding." –Notes from the Doc

----

REALITY - EXPECTATIONS = HAPPINESS

Your happiness is keenly associated with your reality minus your expectations for yourself. A perfect example is one we see with our clients focused on losing weight. A client will set a weight loss goal based on nothing more than a notion, such as, "I want to lose ten pounds in four weeks." In other words, it's often an arbitrary number with an arbitrary deadline. At the end of the four weeks, the client is down eight pounds. Amazing progress, but guess what? They are unhappy because their reality didn't match up with their expectations—ones based on an invented number. Had the goal been six pounds and they had lost eight, would they be any happier? Maybe, but happiness is not based on outcomes alone. Happiness is the art of being content with an otherwise healthy body while embracing the opportunity for support and guidance to achieve a new goal. Sure, dropping the weight may feel good physically, is probably healthier, and it's certainly nice to fit into your pants that had been too tight. We must remember, though, that if one's happiness is conditional, based on this change, it will quickly fade. Instead, we are seeking enduring and lasting happiness.

There's a better way to approach this. First, we need to understand that our weight will not dictate our happiness, so using it as a marker is unwise. We've heard it repeatedly: "I'll be happy when I lose ten pounds." This is not a self-fulfilling prophecy. Even when people succeed in losing weight, their positive emotions are short-lived, and a new, "I'll be happy when…" replaces the earlier condition. The pursuit of an elusive illusion of happiness continues.

A better strategy is to shift your attention to sought-after benefits. Ask yourself: What benefits would the weight loss provide? Am I looking for more capacity to play with my friends and family?

Am I hoping to alleviate worries over health concerns? Do I wish to feel confident in my clothes? All too often, weight loss is just a means to an end, to accomplishing something else. When we realize that, we learn that the number on the scale doesn't matter.

"Most people's assessments show they desire some combination of wanting to learn and share, be understood, make contributions, and be impactful." –Notes from the Doc

----

Second, shifting your focus can be a game-changer. Since happiness is your reality minus your expectations, ensure your expectations are appropriate. The amount of weight you will lose a month from now is difficult to determine. It's tough to set an appropriate expectation based on a number. It is much easier to set expectations on behaviors and actions you can control. You can't control the amount of weight you lose in a day. You can, however, decide whether to work out, to eat a piece of fruit instead of a cookie, and to reach out to a friend instead of isolating yourself. Choices like these aligned with your values lead to sustained success and happiness. This brings us back to being content instead of expecting our days to be packed with peak moments.

CULTIVATING HAPPINESS

Happiness is often viewed as something that happens to us. In other words, we're just passively waiting for good fortune to rain down upon us. And to be fair, moments of happiness can happen randomly. But they are rare and unreliable. We see happiness as more of an active than a passive emotion, as more of a practice than a state. In other words, you possess a measure of control over your own happiness. You can deliberately and intentionally affect your own well-being. You can cultivate your happiness. But just as a farmer cultivates his crops, cultivating your happiness takes effort. The good news is that the reward is well worth it.

To clarify, we're not viewing life through rose-colored glasses. There's no way to escape negative emotions or difficult experiences. Life definitely has its challenges and obstacles, its peaks and valleys. The goal here is to steer our experiences toward the positive end of the emotional spectrum, to spend more time in the realm of happiness, to increase the frequency we participate in happiness. To do that, let's explore several strategies for increasing our happiness.

There will always be problems. What you want is a higher-level problem.

A reset of the negative aspect of making comparisons is required. There are people all over the world who would love to have your "problems." When they play the comparison game, you're at the pinnacle of what they would like to achieve. Your environment is temperature-controlled, your information is delivered wirelessly through the internet, you have access to clean, drinkable water, your waste is miraculously flushed away, your food is healthy and abundant, and your transportation is readily available. You can fly to remote destinations in a matter of hours. Yes, you get to fly!

How mind-blowing is that? Not to mention, diseases that were once fatal are easily inoculated against and infant mortality rates in the developed world are at historical lows. We live in a world our great ancestors could never have imagined.

And, admittedly, we still have problems. But our problems are not those of our ancestors. Our ancestors were worried about scarcity—not having enough food and water to survive. They were focused on securing shelter and avoiding disease. Our ancestors' primary concern was survival.

In contrast, our problems are ones of abundance. Our grocery stores are packed with food. We have clean drinking water at the turn of a tap. There are problems with abundance, such as: paying the electric bill because we want a cool house in the summer. Fretting over the water bill after watering our grass to keep our lawns green. Attaining a healthier weight because food is so readily available. Our problems are not ones of surviving but thriving.

"Good problems" sounds like a contradiction in terms, but many of our current problems fit the bill. We've become desensitized to the relative abundance around us. A moment of reflection brings this back into focus. We can use comparison to our advantage.

"I don't have to chase extraordinary moments to find happiness. It's right in front of me if I'm paying attention and practicing gratitude." –Brene Brown

----

The default setting for the human brain is to focus on the negative, to identify threats, to be alert to deficiencies. For millennia, this negative-oriented outlook kept our species alive. The cave-man who more vigilantly and consistently identified threats in his environment was more apt to live. Keeping watch for tigers in the jungle was necessary for survival. With this in mind, it's easy to see why our brain is programmed to determine our level of safety and be alert to potential threats. We're hardwired to see the problems and develop a numb familiarity to the good things.

"Grateful people are less depressed and experience more positive emotions because of their perspective, not their possessions." –Notes from the Doc

----

But even this hardwiring can be sidestepped. How? With grati-tude. As our natural inclination drives us to dwell on the absence of things in our lives, gratitude steers us back to the vast abun-dance we experience daily.

Gratitude can be practiced in several ways. One option is daily journaling and listing three things you're grateful for. Another op-tion is to practice gratitude when facing a challenging situation. In the midst of such circumstances, pause for a moment to list a few things you are grateful for either on paper or by making a mental note. Gratitude can be incredibly powerful and can dramatically improve your life.

Because each of us has unique wants and desires, you must really think about what makes you happy. This requires daily self-reflection; it will take time and change as you evolve. What makes you happy is something that we can't answer in our book. After basic needs are met, what makes people happy varies and can even be on opposite ends of the spectrum. For example, learning a musical instrument brings some people joy while silent meditation flips the switch for others. Working long, unpredictable hours provides a sense of fulfill- ment for some while others see happiness bloom with a consistent 8–5 schedule. Neither is good or bad, just unique to that individual.

The goal here is to clarify what cultivates happiness for you and no one else. It's best to avoid defaulting to easy answers and com- mon responses. We want the right answers to your unique path. Through introspection and reflection, identify the keys to cultivat- ing your happiness.

"So, please, I implore you to understand yourself and know what makes you tick. Know what makes you happy and find the time to do that. Find your happiness and win."
–Gary Vaynerchuck

So, with each day, each relationship, and every trip or expe- rience start digging deeply into what you enjoyed and what you didn't enjoy. Take time to reflect. That will allow you to make choices aligned with your unique path toward happiness. These reflections and adjustments can become part of your everyday life, creating the level of contentment we all crave.

CHICKEN OR EGG?

Consider these two statements: "People who are really fit must be happy." "The reason people are fit is because they are happy."

Which one is true? Are people happy because they're fit? Or are they fit because they're happy? The answer is both, but that's not the whole story.

Let's look at the first statement, "People who are really fit must be happy." You've probably made this assumption many times and you're partly right. Being physically and mentally fit are most certainly correlated with happiness. Having the capacity to do the things you want to, assuage health concerns, and wear your clothes with confidence can add to your sense of contentment. Fitness is definitely a piece of the happiness puzzle and a valuable asset to your experience of life. However, physical fitness in isolation is rarely enough to make you happy.

The second statement, "The reason people are fit is because they are happy" may seem a bit more surprising, but it contains a measure of truth. The happier you are, the less stressed you are, and stress can wreak havoc on your fitness. As you learned in the chapter on stress, the more stressed you are, the worse your digestive system functions, the more disrupted your sleep becomes and the more junk food you crave and consume. These factors contribute to a lack of fitness.

There's no doubt that being physically and mentally fit are correlated with happiness, which is why it is crucial to identify what fitness looks like for you. Your unique definition and its daily pursuits are the keys to achieving that happiness.

Happiness helps keep stress at bay. Happiness will improve many other areas of your fitness, relationships, and health. It will contribute to your willingness to try new things and not worry about following the herd and emulating everyone else.

Just as being really fit is not the sole catalyst to your happiness, being happy is not the sole catalyst to your fitness, but it is a valuable contributor. Being happy can accelerate your fitness journey and being fit can enhance your happiness.

As we have highlighted in this chapter, happiness isn't a specific weight, body fat percentage, level of strength, or the ability to strike a difficult yoga pose. Happiness is the culmination of our daily actions and thoughts. Happiness, like eating right and being active, must be something we work on every day. This will help you create the lean, healthy, and contented life we all seek.

The table below presents recommendations for increasing happiness. In the ADD column, we propose behaviors to add to your daily activities. In the LIMIT column, we include behaviors to limit in your daily activities.

ADD
List the things and activities that make you happy; do those things.
Schedule time to do something fun with someone close to you.
Plan a vacation or a get-away.
LIMIT
Reduce or eliminate news for a week.
Reduce time spent on social media by 10 minutes per day.
Create a list of people who detract from your happiness and limit time with those people.

For a deeper understanding of these and other strategies, visit TheRedefit.com.

NOTES FROM THE DOC

Recently I saw a social media post requesting that people share how they found work-life balance. Many people commented on how they limit this to get that and say no to this to do that. How is that going for people? Not very well. Unfortunately, despite good intentions, the overuse and incorrect use of the term "work-life balance" has just added one more thing to everyone's I-suck-at-this list. The reason for this is that work-life balance insinuates a tradeoff and the visual often used to represent this is a perfectly level scale. Many of us are not wired that way, nor is that what makes us happy. Most people are not inspired by the idea of carefully scripting out their day and limiting their passions to restricted hours and activities. So, for example, if you are passionate about serving others and you have a job that affords you that opportunity, you may choose to work more because it makes you happy. In this case, there's no need to restrict work hours because work brings you happiness. Or if you love to learn and your job doesn't afford you opportunities to learn, you may choose to limit your work hours and spend your free time reading or traveling. The concept for work-life balance did not come from science indicating that your daily activities and pursuits need to be perfectly balanced. It came from the current mental health crisis many developed countries face. As we are exposed to more options and information, we try to do it all, and if we can't it's because we aren't using the right technology, don't know the right people, or don't work at the right company. There is no such thing as doing it all, and by trying, we are mentally imploding.

"You can't always get what you want, but....you get what you need." –Rolling Stones

----

LIFE'S BUCKETS

The definition of need is something an organism requires to live a healthy life. This is not simply water, food, and shelter. A healthy, happy life also includes mental health. Buying a new piece of trendy clothing or a tech toy may offer a short-lived peak moment, but we do not need these things to be happy. Note Maslow's hierarchy of needs, a theory of motivation in psychology developed by Abraham Maslow. The chart below illustrates the theory.

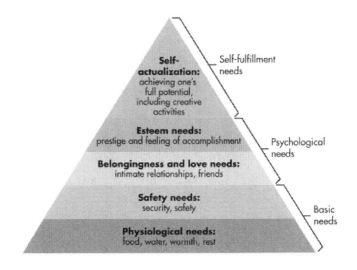

When was the last time these needs were on someone's birthday wish list? Yet once we understand how they can be met in our daily life, we can have a peak life and find true happiness. The problem is when we do not spend time identifying our true needs, we resort to letting our friends, coworkers, and family define happiness for us. We can have it all; we just need to know what that means for us. When we know what life buckets we need and how much of each makes us happy, we can find the right life ratio.

These buckets are functionally the categories of our lives from which we make deposits and withdrawals to lead our lives. This is the other reason that work-life balance is misleading. Work is simply a label to categorize a part of life. For some it's simply a means to an end—to pay for daily living—and for others, it's an expression of their passions and vision. Ideally, it would serve as both. Work is just one of the many buckets in our lives. Unfortunately, lots of people believe that happiness at work is defined by pay, status, and perks. For many of the companies I work with, we do assessments on the employees. The assessments are often designed to help those employees define what they truly value and what makes them happy. Not every assessment can determine this and ideally, people would be able to answer that question. Yet they can't. Most people's assessments show that they desire some combination of wanting to learn and share, be understood, make contributions, and be impactful. Notice the correlation between these desires and the higher rungs in Maslow's hierarchy.

However, most people believe a script that claims the truth is locked behind a deadbolt and they cannot find the proverbial key. If that's the case, we need to pick the lock to get to the truth. The first step is to think about our hierarchy of needs and recognize the life buckets that can meet those needs. For example, not every job is amazing and fulfilling. However, if a job allows you to get your basic needs met, it's serving an important purpose. The challenge comes when we spend 12-hour days just meeting our basic needs and have nothing left for our other needs (this may be necessary at times). Psychologically, we need to be challenged. If your work or home is not challenging you, think about what would challenge you. Would you be inspired by reading about something or somewhere new? What about working on a new physical challenge, like walking a 5k, or acro-yoga? When you spend time with your friends and family, do you feel a sense of belonging and acceptance? If not, consider mixing up your tribe a bit. Or perhaps you work extra hours because co-workers provide a sense of belonging and you feel challenged there. Spend some time with the hierarchy and map out where your needs are being met, and how much time you devote to those areas. They also note the detractors and identify ways to minimize them. You will need to do this repeatedly as circumstances and seasons of our lives change. Working with the hierarchy will help you see that what you need and what you want are aligned. From there you can find your life ratio.

Many varied professional disciplines have sought to define happiness. There is a branch of psychology, called positive psychology, dedicated to identifying the root causes of happiness and methods for achieving it. Most professionals agree that it's a state of being necessary for a healthy lifestyle. The culminating research has suggested several factors or habits associated with happy people. I have highlighted a few here—this is not an exhaustive list—for you to get started on your journey.

Relationships – This is a quality-over-quantity situation. Happy people are thought to have several close relationships that allow them to express themselves and communicate genuine care and commitment. What's key to these relationships is active communicative engagement.

Understanding your Strengths – Studies indicate that happy people have a sense of their strengths (i.e. problem solver, good listener) and purposely use those strengths to meaningfully impact the world around them. This may be through work, family, community or all three.

Acts of Kindness – "It is always better to give than receive" is what parents have told their children for generations. Studies show that this is not just a cultural edict. In fact, we are wired to be happier and less depressed when we try to connect with and support others.

Finding your Fit – There is extensive research on the impact of exercise and food on our mental health and well-being. People have consistently responded to exercise and healthier food choices with less depression and more happiness.

Positive Mindset – This has been a significant area of study in positive psychology. Happy people have been found to have a consistent optimistic perspective. Grateful people are less depressed and experience more positive emotions because of their perspective, not their possessions.

Again, these are just a few of the key characteristics that research suggests contributes significantly to our state of happiness. And, as with most things in life, employing a moderate amount of several of these habits will extend the benefits far more than an excess of one.

We are all unique, so your blend of these habits won't look like anyone else's. However, the next time you are looking for a tribe or reflecting on your needs, evaluate the hierarchy we've presented here, and the habits, and find your personal happy.

CHAPTER 7
RELATIONSHIPS

"No man is an island."—John Donne

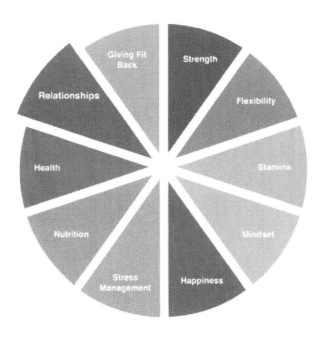

It may not be evident today with the ease of modern conveniences and infrequent life-threatening situations, but we are hardwired to maintain relationships with fellow humans for survival. In today's world, we can have food and other goods delivered to our homes, pay our bills online, work remotely, and all but eliminate face-to-face human interaction. But is this good for us?

Modern advancements like the smartphone and cloud technology and relative miracles such as stem cell research may have revolutionized society, but we must remember they have only recently been introduced. In fact, the World Wide Web is only 28 years old, having first appeared on the scene in 1990. Although it feels like smartphones have been around forever, the first iPhone was released just 12 years ago in 2007. The pace of technology is blistering, but it is very recent in light of millions of years of human evolution.

Our ingrained behaviors, subconscious biases, and underlying drives are hundreds of millennia old. They haven't had a chance to catch up with modern living. If we take a trip down our species' memory lane, removed from the relative opulence and comfort we enjoy daily, we see the necessity for relationships and community. Back in hunter-gatherer days, trust between individuals was necessary for survival. Sharing was a way of life. Some members of the tribe were hunters. Others were gatherers. Still, others protected the little ones. There were those who cooked and those who tended the fire. The many roles necessary for survival were shared by the group which formed a tribe. Life inside the tribe, connected and reliant on others, was still challenging, but much better than a solitary life. In fact, tribe members' survival depended on it.

Could an individual survive outside the tribe? Yes, but the

threats and responsibilities that were mitigated and shared by the tribe would be heaped on the individual. Long-term prospects for survival would shrink. The individuals that built and maintained relationships were the ones who survived to hand down their genes.

And now, here we are, several hundred millennia later. We may live in a world where people can voluntarily isolate themselves by working from home, having all their necessities delivered, and on-line banking. But the hardwiring to connect with fellow humans remains. Despite the technological advances that allow us to isolate ourselves, we're still social creatures. The drive and the accompanying reward are ingrained in our genes.

But, as with our ancestors, not just any relationships will do. We want what they wanted—relationships that enrich our lives, assuage threats, and provide safety and stability. Relationships are an integral part of our lives and have the potential to strongly influence our life experience. They affect your levels of stress and happiness and can help determine your fitness. Your relationships affect your environment and your environment influences your life choices and direction. We must examine these relationships and steer them in a direction that benefits those involved.

We will delve into four areas of relationships: your relationship with yourself, relationships with others, relationship reevaluation, and relationship quality.

"Make sure your worst enemy doesn't live between your ears."
–Laird Hamilton

RELATIONSHIP WITH YOURSELF

Improving your relationship with yourself is the first step in cultivating positive relationships with others. Unfortunately, this aspect of relationships is often overlooked. We can be very hard on ourselves, to the point of it being detrimental to our well-being. Building yourself up is of utmost importance in creating the life and relationships you want. The more you can accept yourself for who you are and what you want, the more others will be able to do the same. You have the most control over your relationship with yourself. As you learn to accept and love yourself, others will follow suit.

Self-love and acceptance are a daily practice. Many people talk more negatively to themselves than they would to their worst enemy. In fact, we often hear people say, "I am not going to put any negativity out there," but they repeatedly allow their inner voice to go negative. There is a place for evaluation and constructive criticism, yet often, we do not differentiate between constructive criticism and negative self-talk.

We must focus on our assets, contributions, and the ways in which we are working to improve ourselves. Something as simple as a gratitude journal is a powerful tool for aligning our inner voice with our goals. Focusing on the relative abundance and opportunity in our lives makes us positive people to be around, which in turn attracts positive people. As with all relationships, the relationship with yourself takes time and requires cultivation.

"Whatever we focus on will grow." —Notes from the Doc

RELATIONSHIPS WITH OTHERS

We touched on the importance of relationships in the chapter on stress management, but in this chapter, we will look at it more deeply. As we've discussed, we've survived as a species through a tribe-like mentality; it's encoded in our DNA. Essentially the only reason we are here today is that our ancestors worked, cooperated, and shared a common goal of survival with others. In the modern era, survival is manageable without a tribe, however, we are alive not just to survive but to thrive.

If you are reading this book, you are likely living at a socioeconomic level in which most of your basic needs are met. It's safe to assume that you ate in the last 24 hours, slept with a roof over your head, had access to clean drinking water, and there isn't a major plague threatening your survival. This last point may be overly dramatic, but it is a reminder that we are extremely fortunate to have so many modern conveniences, such as health care, as well as economic opportunities.

With our basic needs met, we're surviving, but we want more for ourselves. We crave a sense of purpose, belonging, and contentedness. This comes from belonging to the right tribe. Just as in our distant past, the right tribe can help you achieve greater things as compared to going it alone. Doing things only for ourselves isn't likely fulfilling in the long-term and doesn't give us a sense of purpose and belonging we crave. Let's revisit the example we used in the stress section. How would it make you feel to give back, to volunteer at a soup kitchen, and help the less fortunate? If you've never tried volunteering, give it a go. You'll be amazed by the fulfillment and contentment that connecting and supporting humans in need offers you.

And unlike working alone, a tribe also makes it possible to accomplish big tasks. Consider any big company, law enforcement agency, or hospital. Now imagine only one person running any one of these complex organizations. No one person can fulfill all roles. There's too much to do and too much to know. Your tribe can support you in your complex professional endeavors.

"The tribes we belong to significantly impact how we view fitness. This is one of the reasons, in our effort to redefine fitness, we have created an online community—a RedeFit tribe—to encourage and support a healthier lifestyle approach to fitness." –Notes from the Doc

----

This isn't just confined to work; it also applies to fitness. A tribe that exerts positive peer pressure on you can keep you consistently executing behaviors that will move you closer to your goals. A tribe with high expectations can elevate your performance. Modern-day tribes could include a running group, a workout class, or a group of gym-goers who know you. Camaraderie and participation groups can greatly improve your success rate. Wouldn't that be nice?

"Normative conformity often leads to pervasive changes in our behavior and beliefs in ways that we are not cognizant of, yet can contribute to a nagging sense of a lack of fulfillment and even shame." –Notes from the Doc

----

Now think about people sharing similar struggles, going on the same journey, and working alongside you. That support, the security of knowing there is someone there for you will lead to greater success. That is the tribe we are looking for. That's another reason we created our online platform—so like-minded people could meet and connect to share their experiences on their fitness journeys.

RELATIONSHIP REEVALUATION

Peer pressure and expectations are double-edged swords. Positive peer pressure and higher expectations can elevate us. They can drive us to become better versions of ourselves. Unfortunately, the converse is also true. Negative peer pressure and lower expectations can drag us back down to baseline or even lower.

One of the most difficult relationship conversations we have with clients is when we discuss the people in their lives who might not be right for them as they move toward health and fitness. Imagine you are working hard to improve your fitness and you have a long-time "friend" who is constantly giving you a hard time for your efforts. Their remarks include things like, "Live a little" or "One dessert won't hurt you" or "Come on, have a little fun." Your friend is trying to sabotage your success, because you are trying to improve in an area while your friend is not, triggering your friend's guilt or the feeling of being left out. The friend isn't necessarily being malicious but may be operating on a subconscious level and likely out of fear. After all, this departure from former behaviors signals that you are leaving your friend's tribe.

At this point, you are at a crossroads. Have a serious conversation with your friend and see if they can be supportive. If not, you will choose to spend far less time with that friend. This isn't an easy conversation but one that is needed. You'll be grateful you did in the long-term. This can be challenging, especially if it is your best friend from college, sibling, or your significant other, which is the most difficult. The key is being open and honest, letting them know how you feel when they make comments or behave in a way that negatively affects you. It is important to let them know how much their relationship means to you. Explain how you want to maintain and grow that relationship, which includes being supportive of healthy habits.

Such conversations can let you know when a relationship has run its course. That's okay. Each of us is on our own unique path. The good news is these conversations can deepen relationships and add meaning. And you can exert some positive peer pressure on those close to you.

The path to fitness can be very difficult without the support of others. Making sure you are spending a significant amount of time with positive support is critical to your long-term success.

With the adoption of new healthy habits, this is a great opportunity to make new friends with a common mindset. You might find them in a workout group, a yoga class, or while running. We thrive when keeping the company of like-minded people. When you can surround yourself with people with similar goals and values, you win.

Positive and supportive relationships start with you accepting yourself for who you are and who you really want to be.

RELATIONSHIP QUALITY

In our modern era with social media, digital devices at our side, and gyms where every workout is a competition, it's easy to have lots of "friends." Proximity shouldn't be the reason you choose your circle of friends. Make sure they share common values and fitness goals. The key here is quality over quantity. Which friends are bringing you joy, which ones are supportive of your fitness journey, and which ones can you rely on when you're down? They need to support you and you need to support them. Those are the ones that need your attention. To show up for them, ensure you are bringing joy to their life, encouraging them in their journey, and be supportive when they are down. This builds the strong tribe you seek. This supports your fit body and fit mind.

Positive and supportive relationships with yourself and others are paramount for your success on your fitness journey. It starts with you accepting yourself for who you are and who you really want to be, not what you think others want. Then you reevaluate your current social circle and nurture your best relationships or create new ones to shape the tribe that will help you on your journey.

The following table presents recommendations for improving relationships. In the ADD column, we propose behaviors to add to your daily activities. In the LIMIT column, we include behaviors to limit in your daily activities.

ADD
List 3 things you like about yourself.
Send a thank you note to someone who impacted you.
Have a cell phone-free meal with someone close to you.

LIMIT
Refrain from comparing yourself to others.
Limit eating out with friends who don't eat healthy.
Avoid gossiping.

For a deeper understanding of these and other strategies, visit TheRedefit.com.

NOTES FROM THE DOC

Do you recall a time as a teenager when you pursued a special boy or girl for a friendship or a relationship? Or perhaps there was a time when you wanted to be part of a group of children at school. Reflect on your behaviors. What did you do? Most likely it was some combination of: follow them around, conveniently be in the same place and time, dress in a way you thought they might like or think was cool, pretend to like the music they liked but you secretly hated. Or maybe you did something you knew was stupid, but they said it was cool. The list goes on—right? Thank goodness our teenage years are over, and we do not feel the need to engage in those kinds of behaviors anymore…or do we?

Many times, in this book we have said that humans are wired to want to belong to a tribe of sorts: with others like us, who accept us, and with whom we can safely explore and strive together to reach our goals. A lot of good can come from the tribe mentality. However, there are times when the tribe mentality can get us in trouble. This often results from what psychologists and sociologists call social conformity. Social conformity simply represents changes in one's behavior or beliefs as a result of social influence in order to fit in with a group.

In a now popular study among psychologists conducted by Solomon Asch, participants were asked to evaluate and compare the length of several lines placed on two cards. All but one participant were actors who purposely gave an obviously incorrect answer. Asch measured how many times the actual participants conformed to the group answer. About 75 percent did so at least one time and only about 25 percent never conformed. When those that did conform were asked why, they indicated one of two reasons—

to fit in with the group, or because they felt they must have been missing something since everyone else was so confident about their answers. These are examples of normative and informational conformity, respectively.

NORMATIVE CONFORMITY

Normative conformity is the result of wanting to be liked or accepted. For those who tend to be more social and enjoy being known and included, being liked in a group is important. For those who do not want to stand out and simply want to be part of a team or group, being accepted is the goal. Again, our thoughts turn to teenagers and peer pressure. This is because teens often have underdeveloped identities and are not sure who should be in their tribe. Additionally, as they develop, their desires and personalities continue to evolve (especially as the hormones loosen their grip) and so we see them rotate through various tribes. They need to sample to see what feels right.

However, it's not just teenagers that are affected; it's all of us. When was the last time you had dinner with friends and a dish or two was not very tasty? You ate silently while reminding yourself of the adage, "If you do not have something nice to say, do not say anything." But then someone piped in about how amazing the dishes tasted, and then several more people. After an awkward pause, did you also compliment it? Have you ever reluctantly engaged in a standing ovation for a mediocre performance after it became uncomfortable to be the only person sitting? We are taught these normative conformity behaviors from an early age—sometimes simply referred to as "manners." We are encouraged to be positive and not the buzzkill of an event or interaction. As such we constantly weigh our contributions and filter ourselves. To some degree, this is part of being in a tribe. However, normative conformity often leads to pervasive changes in our behavior and even our beliefs in ways that we are not cognizant of yet can contribute to a nagging sense of a lack of fulfillment and even shame. These tendencies toward conformity can impact all aspects of our lives, including moral values, how we vote in elections, where and how we live, and what we wear.

Think about a time you were with family or friends and you said "no" to a second helping or chose a healthy alternative and you were teased or harassed as being to uptight, a health nut or a buzzkill. Perhaps it was the time when you declined an invitation to go shopping or watch a game in lieu of working out. Were you told that you could work out another time? Or perhaps someone said, "What will missing one workout do?" How did you respond? Did you skip your workout? Do you stop eating healthily in front of certain people or in certain situations to avoid this? Have there been times you were the one dishing out the teasing or pressure to conform? Now of course, clearly there is a time and place for getting harassed by your friends or joining in an activity that our friends and family are doing that we might not typically do. In moderation, this is psychologically a healthy thing for us and our relationships. However, the challenge arises when we do not realize how much, how often, and how deviant the group expectations are from what actually makes us happy and fulfilled. This is why we stress in this chapter to first work on your relationship with yourself. What do you need to challenge yourself, to feed your soul, and to be the best you for achieving your goals at this moment and for the future? Once you can articulate the story of you, then you can evaluate the other relationships in your life to assess what groups you will thrive in and under what conditions.

INFORMATIONAL INFLUENCE

As I mentioned earlier, in the famous study by Asch, there is a second reason people conform: the assumption that everyone else has information we don't. This is why people often vote along party lines but may be hard-pressed to articulate specifics about a candidate. If the party nominated a given candidate, they must have a good reason for doing so. Have you ever researched a product, were all set to buy it, but then your friends indicated they had bought a different one? If so, you probably did the calculation that if most of your friends chose that product, it must be good despite your research to the contrary. This phenomenon is called informational influence and occurs when the correct behavior mode is not clear, and people look to others for cues, assuming the actions of the masses indicate appropriateness. This is more commonly referred to as a "herd mentality."

When the masses are correct, the herd mentality may be beneficial. Think about social movements in history that have impacted positive and significant change. Unfortunately, because of the desire to fit in, groups of people will act together even in the absence of little rational proof. Most of us have heard about individuals leading large groups into chaos or harm's way resulting in political and humanitarian atrocities. We are most susceptible to this phenomenon when those leading are revered and viewed as knowledgeable. We have seen the herd mentality influence social media and health and fitness trends. For instance, weren't many of us disappointed to find out holding a weight that vibrates will do nothing for us other than make us feel like human gelatin? Or that eating chocolate and drinking wine daily is not actually the recipe for improved health? Note, I said disappointed. I did not say surprised. Because we weren't surprised, we always knew that these tools and diets defied basic logic, yet the ads and confident spokespeople reminded us that everyone was buying them and getting amazing results. Despite our better judgment, we assume we are missing information and so they must be right in their claims.

SOCIAL CONFORMITY AND SOCIAL MEDIA

The advent of the internet and social media has dramatically improved access to more and varied tribes. Pictures, videos, and text shared on social media offer an endless platform for connecting and getting information. It has also accelerated our potential to be sucked into both normative and informational conformity; to be accepted and liked and to make sure we are not missing anything. The fear of missing out (FOMO) has become a widespread phenomenon. To debate, the pros and cons of the information age, feel free to go to the web, where such a debate rages endlessly. Meanwhile, for the purposes of this chapter, I want to highlight how this phenomenon translates into shaming and specifically impacts our daily fit journey.

Shaming has been around as long as humans have graced the planet. There are many terms for it and it comes in many forms. It is a psychological form of "shine and tarnish." To make myself shine, I will tarnish you. A new penny is very shiny compared to an old penny but not very shiny compared to a crystal. There is an exhaustive list of reasons people feel the need to tarnish others, including an effort to appear more impressive or better looking.

The goal here is to help you learn how to recognize it in yourself and others and how to think about it differently.

Cultural and societal practices often dictate what is considered beautiful or appropriate. It varies by gender and ethnicity and can even be influenced by fashion trends. The more we are exposed to these values, the more likely we are to incorporate them into the definition of beauty and what makes others attractive or healthy. As such, the tribes we belong to significantly impact how we view fitness. This is one of the reasons in our effort to redefine fitness, we have created an online community—a RedeFit tribe—to encourage and support a healthier lifestyle approach to fitness. However, when those we follow on social media, spend time with, and admire judge or criticize others different from them, it increases the likelihood that we will subscribe to those same perspectives and behaviors.

Think back to the examples of peer pressure. If you have ever changed your eating or activities around others because of their comments, you most likely have been shamed for making healthy choices. Some call this fit shaming. Have you ever called someone a couch potato? Was that a compliment or a judgment? Is it leading by example, or is it shine and tarnish? Furthermore, on your fitness journey, when you are fit-shamed, how do you let it affect you?

The *story of you* that I referenced earlier is essential. What do you care about, what makes you happy and what challenges you to be a better you? What tribes support those behaviors? Can you use social media to connect with those people? Will this tribe offer encouragement, share strategies to promote your goals, provide resources for responding to shaming, and can you trust them to do the research too on what is effective for the changes you want to make?

Chapter 8
Nutrition

"People often attribute a lack of success on the healthy eating journey to a lack of motivation or willpower. Although discipline and commitment to a healthy lifestyle are required, the culprit is usually emotional eating." –Notes from the Doc

----

Of all the aspects of comprehensive fitness, nutrition is possibly the most confusing. It seems like there's a new miracle diet unveiled every other week with claims to overhaul your health and wellness. Or that the latest and greatest nutrition fad is taking the world by storm and blowing up social media. Or that a revolutionary superfood is making a splash in popular magazines, online, and every media outlet. It's overwhelming and exhausting to keep up. Just when you've embraced one fad, another one overtakes it and you have to recalibrate.

Compounding the confusion, nutrition is a topic with the potential to be as heated as religion and politics. We all know people who have solidified their views on nutrition, espouse them as if they were gospel, and resist other viewpoints. With so many options and zealous disciples of these various approaches, it's no wonder many of us wrestle with our nutrition.

It doesn't have to be like this. It's time to understand nutrition so you can harness it as one of your most powerful tools in achieving the look, vitality, and health you desire. This chapter will not only bring you clarity but will illustrate that good nutrition doesn't have to be boring or an experience of monkish self-deprivation. Good nutrition can be exciting, delicious, and include occasional treats.

TWO SIDES OF A COIN: TECHNICAL AND EMOTIONAL

Proper nutrition is a smart balance of two factors—technical and emotional. The technical side of nutrition includes variables such as calories, macronutrients, micronutrients, timing, and food quality. Most approaches emphasize the technical aspect of nutrition. And, although this must be addressed, the focus on the technical side often neglects the emotional side of proper nutrition. The emotional side includes elements such as stress, environment, and behavioral tendencies.

Let's start with an overview before exploring both topics in detail. In the big picture, how do most diets attempt to help you achieve and maintain a healthy weight? They put you at a smart caloric intake. Simple—right? Weight loss versus weight gain is easy math. If more energy (calories in this case) is coming in than going out, weight gain occurs. If more energy is going out than coming in, weight loss occurs.

Establishing a smart caloric intake from primarily whole food (unprocessed and unrefined) sources is the cornerstone to proper nutrition. So, since achieving and maintaining a healthy body weight is as simple as smart caloric intake, then the question remains: why do most diets **not** work?

The answer is simple. Most diets restrict the dieter to the point of rebellion. They make consistency nearly impossible. They rely on willpower in the short-term and when that fails, they send us into a downward spiral of binging on ice cream, cookies, chocolate, and other treats within arm's reach. In short, they ignore the emotional side of nutrition.

Let's look at an example to illustrate this point. Imagine a diet of nothing but chicken and broccoli. (To be clear, we are not advocating this.) Would a person lose weight with this approach? Most likely. It's so restrictive that a caloric deficit would result. And, as you read earlier, a caloric deficit leads to weight loss. But this approach is shortsighted. And only addressing the technical side of nutrition is a mistake. The emotional side must get equal, if not more, attention. From an emotional perspective, would you be able to sustain this approach long enough to see the weight loss? Probably not, because it is boring, monotonous, and takes the joy out of food. In other words, it's nearly impossible to sustain.

"When we sabotage ourselves so brilliantly—especially in the eating department—this is typically emotional eating. In essence, we are self-medicating." –Notes from the Doc

----

Food is our fuel and provides the nutritional building blocks we need to survive and thrive. Nutrition is a tool to attain and maintain the body and vitality we want. But that's not the whole story. Food is delicious, brings us joy, and provides a means for social interaction. Food is tied to emotions—both central to our celebrations and an outlet for our stress. Any plan that tries to achieve the technical side of nutrition without addressing the emotional side is tough to implement and impossible to sustain. The RedeFit Model is a holistic approach that addresses both the technical and the emotional sides tied to good nutrition while tailoring the approach to your needs and goals.

DEEPER DIVE: THE EMOTIONAL SIDE

In this section, we will give you immediately implementable tools to help you understand yourself and navigate the emotional side of nutrition. There are innumerable fitness plans that consist of eating certain foods, working out a certain way, or setting up specific habits, but if they aren't tailored to how you are individually wired then it will be extremely difficult to create consistency and the results you're striving for.

The next few sections will introduce different frameworks that will help you understand yourself, your past behaviors and give you the knowledge to steer your actions and environment to your advantage.

Moderate Indulger or Abstainer

We've all heard the advice "moderation is key." Although well-intentioned, it only works for people who can indulge moderately. Consider the mindset of an alcoholic. Should that person's goal be a little alcohol every day? Or do you think abstaining from alcohol would be best? Of course, an alcoholic can't control their impulses so must abstain from alcohol.

Most people fall into one of two major categories: moderate indulger or abstainer. A moderate indulger is satisfied with a small amount of food or drink—someone who can control the total amount consumed and finds less pleasure if they have more. For example, a moderate indulger can eat just one square of chocolate candy bar each day, making it last for a week or more. The next type—abstainers—marvel at moderate indulgers and their self-control.

An abstainer is someone who must stay away from an indulgence completely or at least have limited access to the total amount because this person can't control their impulses to enjoy a treat. If we revisit our chocolate bar example, we would see the abstainer have the same good intentions as the moderate indulger—just one square of chocolate each day. Moments later, the abstainer would eat the entire bar in one sitting.

This is not passing judgment on abstainers or shaming them for their apparent lack of willpower. Full disclosure: we're abstainers. Instead, this is to provide insight to set you up for success.

You're probably nodding your head, strongly identifying as either a moderate indulger or an abstainer. If you're still unsure, take a moment to reflect on your past behaviors and you'll see one pattern more strongly expressed. Take note of which category you fall into. Neither one is better than the other, but the self-knowledge will help you create a sustainable lifestyle.

So now that you've identified with one of these two categories, what should you do? If you are a moderate indulger, it's safe to keep your minor indulgence in your home if it's an occasional treat. Your natural tendencies allow for this treat in your environment without it derailing you.

"Researchers suggest that when stressed we crave high-fat high-sugar foods that chemically reduce the stress response hormones and increase serotonin to calm the brain." –Notes from the Doc

----

If you're an abstainer, don't keep your special treat around. Temptations in close proximity will not set up your environment for success. This doesn't mean no treats ever again; it just means you need to approach it differently. If you want to keep the treat in your life, plan for it, treat yourself on special occasions, and perhaps share it with a loved one. Your goal is to reduce the frequency of those experiences. This will allow you to enjoy it without it being detrimental to your goals. Situations at work or in social settings may arise where this becomes more difficult but having a plan of staying away completely is typically easier as an abstainer than attempting to moderately indulge.

Stress Over- or Under-Eating

Another area that will offer insight into is your response to stress. Most of us are familiar with how stress alters eating patterns. Some people deal with stress by over-consuming food, whereas others cope by under-consuming food. With a brief glance at your past behaviors, you'll be able to identify which pattern characterizes you.

If you're a stress overeater, the default stress-reliever is food. Food is easily accessible and quickly rewarding. So, stress over-eaters must find other ways to reduce stresses that are non-food related and healthily sustainable. A positive replacement could be working out, walking, meditating, playing an instrument, listening to music, or going for a run. Find an activity that works for you and choose that as your stress-reliever.

If you under-eat when stressed, you must be aware of skipping meals, being undernourished, and stressing your body by under-eating. It's important to be aware of this pattern and to have a plan for food that is accessible and easy to eat when you're stressed, such as a shake, fruit, or a protein bar. This will help you stay on track with your nutrition and not create more stress.

Are You a Planner or an Impulsive?

When you think about prepping food on a Sunday afternoon for the week, does it feel like a breeze or an onerous chore? If you said it was a breeze, you're a planner. If a chore, you're more impulsive. Planners have a leg up because they naturally gravitate toward having their food prepped. As you can imagine, planning for and preparing food is typically the best approach.

But, impulsives, take heart. You can still be successful. The power here comes from the awareness of your natural tendencies. You just need to be familiar with your options. It is important to know what is available if you need something last minute. Ask yourself, *what can I order and have delivered, or pick up, that's still real food?* Once you have your go-to options, you can still stick with the plan and not be too strict with it. You will be true to yourself; your impulsive nature will have the freedom to express itself.

Again, take a moment to note your tendencies. Are you a moderate indulger or an abstainer? A stress over-eater or under-eater? A planner or an impulsive? Insight into your nature will support you in shaping your behaviors and environment to achieve your goals. Now, let's take a look at the technical side of things.

THE TECHNICAL BIG PICTURE

To ensure that you're not overwhelmed by the technical details of nutrition, we're going to implement them in a systematic, measured way to set you up for success.

The big picture guidelines for proper nutrition include the categories, associated amounts, and examples displayed in the following table.

Category	Amount	Examples
Water	Min ½ x bodyweight in ounces of water per day	
Protein	½ x bodyweight to 3/4 x bodyweight in grams per day (7g = approximately 1oz lean meat)	Chicken, egg whites, beef, whey, turkey
Fat	½ x bodyweight in grams per day	Nuts, avocado, egg yolk, butter, cheese
Vegetables	As much as you can eat, ideally with every meal	Spinach, broccoli, cauliflower, beets
Fruit	1 to 2 pieces a day. More if you are lean and active	Blueberries, blackberries, banana, orange, apple
Other Carbohydrates	Only needed if you are lean and active	Rice, oatmeal, grains, fruit juice

If these guidelines are followed, you will get great results. But we're not going to jump into the deep end of the pool with this plan because that would lead to replicating many of the problems with the standard approach. Instead, we're going to take manageable steps so as not to overwhelm you. The RedeFit Model will provide incremental steps designed to be implementable in your daily routines, sustainable so you can achieve and maintain your progress, and specifically tailored to set you up for success. And we're going to begin with a revolutionary tactic.

START BY ADDING

We collectively sigh when we hear the word "diet." If you think of a diet, you think deprivation—right? Your mind anticipates all the restrictions that will accompany your diet. That's because the standard approach is based on avoidance and deprivation, and it depletes willpower. It's time to flip that idea on its head. After all, it hasn't worked.

What if instead we start by adding food? You read that right. We start by *adding*. "But I'm reading this book to *lose* weight!" you're thinking. Stay with us. For too long, many of us have tried to get the body of our dreams by omitting. You've heard the line: *don't think of a pink elephant.* Great, now you're thinking of a pink elephant—right? That's the same approach as the standard diet: *don't eat ice cream, cookies, or your favorite treat.* What are you thinking of now? The very food you're supposed to be avoiding. That's not a recipe for success.

We don't concern ourselves initially with deprivation, but *inclusion.* That means asking, *what is not in my daily nutrition that needs to be?* We start by adding healthy, nutritious options and go from there. Why? Because it requires monumentally less willpower and decision-making. Because it doesn't leave you with a sense of deprivation. And because it changes your focus. It sets you up for success. And the inclusion of healthy, goal-supporting foods eventually displaces unhealthy, goal-sabotaging foods.

Let's, once again, turn to the big picture guidelines we introduced earlier.

Category	Amount	Examples
Water	Min ½ x bodyweight in ounces of water per day	
Protein	½ x bodyweight to 3/4 x bodyweight in grams per day (7g = approximately 1oz lean meat)	Chicken, egg whites, beef, whey, turkey
Fat	½ x bodyweight in grams per day	Nuts, avocado, egg yolk, butter, cheese
Vegetables	As much as you can eat, ideally with every meal	Spinach, broccoli, cauliflower, beets
Fruit	1 to 2 pieces a day. More if you are lean and active	Blueberries, blackberries, banana, orange, apple
Other Carbohydrates	Only needed if you are lean and active	Rice, oatmeal, grains, fruit juice

Keep it simple. With each meal think: *where is my protein source, where is my fat source, where are my vegetables, and do I have enough water?* Imagine a plate and think of it as ¾ full of vegetables and the rest filled with ¼ protein and a portion of fat. That portion could be something like a piece of steak or a chicken breast with avocado. Including healthy food will naturally displace the less healthy options.

The table below presents recommendations for improving your nutrition. In the ADD column, we propose behaviors to add to your daily activities. In the LIMIT column, we include behaviors to limit in your daily activities.

ADD
Increase the amount of daily protein.
Consistently include veggies in your diet.
Increase your water daily water intake.
LIMIT
Reduce the amount of high caloric snacking.
Limit intake of high calorie drinks.
Avoid excessive dining out.

For a deeper understanding of these and other strategies, visit TheRedefit.com

NOTES FROM THE DOC

People often attribute a lack of success on the healthy eating journey to a lack of motivation or willpower. Although discipline and commitment to a healthy lifestyle are required, typically the culprit is *emotional eating*. Think about the times when you have committed to changing your eating habits, been planful, and excited to do so. Next, consider the times you were seeing results, weight loss, increased energy and having less pain. And yet in a flash you not only fell off the wagon, but it stopped and backed over you. You didn't see it coming and were amazed at how quickly and fervently you lost control and found yourself fasting all day and then bingeing at night. Or perhaps you grabbed a carton of ice cream or family size bag of chips and finished them off in one sitting. If this still sounds like a willpower issue to you, ask yourself if this happens with anything else. Do you ever take a test, know every answer and then mid-way choose the wrong answers on purpose? Have you ever played a game, found yourself on a major winning streak, and then purposefully lost? Willpower and motivation are required to start something, but when we sabotage ourselves so brilliantly–especially in the eating department—this is typically emotional eating. In essence, we are self-medicating.

COGNITIVE RESTLESSNESS

We live in a society that promotes multi-tasking and high rates of productivity and busyness. Our modern brains are wired for engagement in satisfying activities and when we do not get it, we feel uneasy, even bored. [1] When we do not have a process for being comfortably calm, (see Chapter 4 on Mindset) we seek stimulation.

Most of us have either experienced or heard of people who do their best thinking in the shower, while running, or on a long drive. Research indicates that this is likely the result of a three-part equation. First, we tend to be the most cognitively creative when the decision-making center of our brain is relaxed, allowing for other parts of our brain that are less censored and emotionally responsive to be highly engaged. Second, when we relax or exercise, dopamine is released which is linked to higher levels of creativity. And finally, we need distraction. Easy, habitual tasks distract our brain from the ineffective solutions we may have been pondering and allows the brain to better free-associate for more effective solutions [2]. While running and showering seem to be productive approaches for a creative energy release, we are more prone to self-medicate with food to generate this energy through eating. This is especially true for those in developed countries where food is plentiful. People who are required to sit for long periods of time doing daily routine work, solving problems, or being creative may overeat while they are working to achieve this stimulation in order to cognitively engage.

It's so easy to munch on potato chips or suck down a high-sugar coffee drink while working. These mindless habits provide oral stimulation to promote cognitive engagement. Grasping this phenomenon helps us understand that *just stop snacking* won't work long-term since the cognitive need remains. But we can have a better plan and replace these habits appropriately. Replacing chips with a handful of almonds, air-popped popcorn, or other healthier snacks that take time to chew can dramatically change sugar and caloric intake. (Note: I said chew, which is why the usefulness of replacement shakes—a popular snack at work—can often be short-lived.) Additionally, healthier snacks will also maintain a level of cognitive energy as opposed to the crashes triggered by sugary and salty snacks. Over time reducing snacking and replacing snacks with breaks where you take a quick walk around the office or outside can provide much improved cognitive processing.

SOCIAL-EMOTIONAL EATING

Throughout this book, we emphasize that the people you surround yourself with are vitally important to your overall physical and emotional health. The reality is few of us have the luxury to hand-pick who we spend time with each day. However, we can be mindful of who we choose for given activities and our value to the group. Again, let's start with understanding and then adjusting.

Humans are wired to belong to a tribe or a gang. Sharing food is an important cultural tradition that enables us to connect with others. We know community and connection promote longevity and health. The emotions of belonging, connection, and acceptance can influence how we eat in a group and the choices we make. We don't need to ditch our friends because we want to change our lifestyle, but we do need to understand how our mini-tribes fit in our lives and be open to joining other mini-tribes that support what we value. To do this we must understand who we want to be when socializing with others.

Social-emotional eating can look very different for people based on their personality type. Knowing and evaluating yourself is highly effective in recognizing and curbing this phenomenon. For example, if you like to stay busy tinkering on a project, working in the yard, playing games, or you simply can't sit still, attending sit-and-talk social gatherings can make you restless. You might even feel physically trapped, regardless of how much you enjoy the company. If the conversation is not highly stimulating, cognitive stimulation is at a deficit. If there is food around, especially snack food, it's extremely easy to use that to stimulate your senses or to avoid focusing on negative or uncomfortable conversations. Being mindful of this can help you cultivate healthier habits. Consider bringing healthy snacks to the gatherings. And avoid being physically trapped, stay on the perimeter, take small breaks to get a drink, use the restroom (even as an excuse to take a short walk), and encourage stimulating games or conversation.

SELF-SOOTHING EATING

Most of us are familiar with the term "comfort foods." They tend to represent something from our culture or upbringing and are often foods that are higher in carbs and fat. When paired with a positive emotion or memory we can easily use these foods to self-soothe emotional stressors or voids. To increase our awareness of this type of emotional eating, we need to understand these foods and what they represent. For example, you tell everyone that *no one* makes garlic mashed potatoes better than your grandma. Others agree they're good but say they prefer their mother's recipe. Their opinions are not as important as the emotions paired with your favorite comfort food. Do those mashed potatoes represent belonging, value, or even safety? Was your grandma a special person in your life? While mashed potatoes may bring you comfort, it's important to remember they are high in carbohydrates and calories and should be eaten in moderation.

Are you self-soothing by snacking on the couch in front of the TV because you are lonely and it's nice to connect with the characters in your special show? Are you having an extra glass of wine at the end of the day because you work very hard and wine is your validation? In other words, you work hard, you can afford it, and you deserve it. No one would subscribe to the idea that we should stop having these emotions. Yet all too often on New Year's Day, we tell ourselves we are going to stop eating our favorite comfort food, or not drink wine anymore, inadvertently creating a sense of emotional deprivation. Hence, we go from "all in" to the "screw it" phase (See Chapter 3). A bit of mindfulness and exploration of what need our excessive behavior is fulfilling is essential to modifying it or replacing it. If that nice bottle of wine is serving as the "I worked hard treat," consider replacing it with a nice carafe that holds one glass at a time. Then you will extend the bottle of wine for the whole week as opposed to a bottle a night. Every time you pour a little wine into the carafe, you can feel special and deserving of a treat. If your favorite TV shows are filling a void of belonging, decide which show is your favorite and keep just one. Then find a book club or a volleyball league to join. Or identify a friend or family member to call and chat or play cards with instead of eating and watching more television.

STRESS EATING

As we discuss in our stress chapter, our bodies physiologically respond to our daily stressors. Although our stressors are no longer related to hunting and basic survival, our body still responds similarly, engaging in fight-flight mode, to handle what may come at us—large or small. When in this state, it is easy to seek out things that will give us more energy. Researchers suggest that when stressed, we crave high-fat high-sugar foods that chemically reduce the stress response hormones and increase the serotonin—effectively calming the brain. Applying the same model of understanding/replacing used for the other types of emotional eating will also serve you well with stress eating.

Stress can be long-term and hard to pinpoint, or it can be immediate, front and center. Obviously reducing stress is important but also finding other, long-term sources of more proactive and healthy ways to calm our brains is key. This may include meditating to start your day, more actively planning for time spent on hobbies and friends or engaging in regular exercise like hikes or walks to increase your stamina, overall energy, and sense of calm. Knowing yourself and what allows you to relax and pairing that with playful moments to counterbalance daily stress is essential.

DEPRESSED EATING

Appetite and depression both originate in the limbic system of the brain [3]. As such, we often see a correlation between depression and under- or over-eating. When the appetite is affected by a low mood, depression or anxiety, eating habits can be disrupted. Furthermore, those being treated with medication for depression can also experience drug side effects that impact appetite. Chronic or significant depression (impacting day-to-day functioning) should be monitored by a medical professional. Temporary or momentary depression is experienced by most people in their lives due to events or experiences. Quite often unplanned appetite and weight change can be a sign that we are not coping optimally. Being aware and monitoring this is essential to moderate the impact, as is support from family and friends, change of environment, or medical attention.

There are countless categories of emotional eating with many associated emotions. Evaluating our habits, and most importantly our emotions will greatly assist us in identifying the lifestyle changes that will work the best for our individual needs. We are emotional creatures and all too often we hear that we need to "stop emotional eating." And while that advice may be good-intentioned, it stops short of delivering the input we need to change our emotional eating habits. Most people would benefit from a better understanding of their emotions and having a plan to acknowledge and process those emotions. Eating may be a part of that; the key is to be mindful of how this need can be approached in a healthy long-term way.

Chapter 9
Health

"The greatest wealth is health." – *Virgil*

Health is something we all want, but it can be challenging to know what we're chasing when we pursue it. Health often hovers below our conscious appreciation. Only in its absence do we notice how essential to life it is. When we're sick or injured we promise ourselves: *when I am healthy again, I'm really going to appreciate it.* But after we've recovered or healed, we forget to cherish every minute of wellness.

Here's an example to illustrate the way in which health dramatically impacts our life experiences. Imagine a vacation during which you're healthy and strong. You are healthy and fit enough to do all the things you dreamed of while anticipating your vacation. Perhaps you're vacationing at a beach where you can swim, snorkel, kayak, and maybe even try surfing. It's refreshing and recharging—just what the doctor ordered.

Now imagine the same vacation with compromised health. Perhaps you caught the flu on the plane to your vacation destination and you're spending most of your time in the hotel room with a fever and nauseated, wishing you were home. Or maybe you're injured, and you have restricted mobility, which limits what you can do. It's draining, exhausting, and demoralizing. You had been looking forward to your vacation for months. It's the same vacation but with very different outcomes dictated by health and fitness.

It can be helpful to think of health as analogous to your computer's operating system. Your operating system is the platform that supports all the programs and apps you're using. It quietly hums along in the background making everything you do on your computer possible. While you work, enjoy entertainment, and learn at the convenience of your keyboard, your operating system is busy juggling the many tasks you're demanding of your computer. You rarely if ever notice it, that is, until there's a problem with it. Then all the productivity, education, and fun that your operating system supported grinds to a halt.

Health is the very platform your life depends on. It is your foundation for living a full and meaningful life.

The same is true of health. Health is the platform that supports our experiences, quietly humming along until it's disrupted by an illness, a new diagnosis, or an injury. When that happens, it drastically impacts our experiences and our capabilities. Then we become acutely aware of the importance of health and the fact that we took it for granted until it was taken away.

In this chapter, we'll present proactive steps for improving your health. It's critical to understand the importance of health before your health deteriorates. Instead of being reactive, we're going to get out ahead of this.

REDEFINING HEALTHY

How do we optimize our physical operating system? First, we need to appreciate health and the factors that impact it. Health is defined as being free of injury or illness. While that definition is a good start, it doesn't go far enough. We must expand the definition of health.

How would you describe a healthy person? It's doubtful that your answer would be as dry as "free from injury or illness." You probably think of characteristics like energetic, vibrant, resilient, and capable; a person who possesses a sense of well-being.

Too often good health is sacrificed for a short-term goal or a pleasure-seeking activity.

These ideas are truer to the notion of health that we're all aiming for—a spirited and capable body, free from injury or illness that supports our work, passions, and experiences. So, why is good health so challenging if it's something that's clearly essential for living a full life?

Too often good health is sacrificed for a short-term goal or a pleasure-seeking activity. Imagine the extreme dieter or someone who follows a quick-fix weight-loss solution. In the short-term, they may lose weight, but in the long-term, it is likely that they will gain it back—maybe even adding some extra pounds. Or imagine an extreme runner or competitive lifter who tends to over-train for a competition. Carried away by their enthusiasm, they often injure themselves from doing too much too fast while neglecting recovery. These individuals focus on the short-term without giving their health its due attention.

Now consider another extreme. Picture the person who eats only for short-term satisfaction— deliciously rich meals high in calories, or someone who won't do any physical activity because other activities, like watching TV, are easier. We're all aware that actions have consequences and yet people make choices that compromise their health anyway.

"Goal setting is highly correlated with delayed gratification and overall success." –Notes from the Doc

----

Both examples are people focused on short-term gratification. If we return to our analogy of a computer's operating system, these examples would be akin to downloading an app that provided instant entertainment but then plagued your computer with pop-ups, push notifications, and advertisements. The productivity, efficiency, and entertainment your computer once offered are interrupted and diminished.

When it comes to our health, we need to consider how present decisions will affect us in the long-term. Achieving and maintaining your health is an ongoing process. So, how do we keep our aim true? We focus on our expanded definition of health.

MEASURING HEALTH

As stated earlier, our definition of health includes "free from injury or illness" and extends beyond that to encompass the vitality and capacity we want in our lives. Both facets of our definition must be addressed.

If we want to address the idea of "freedom from injury or illness," we can turn to modern medicine. Lab tests and health markers offer great insight. Being tested regularly enables you to peek under your hood to get an idea of healthy or unhealthy trends in your bloodwork and allows for early detection of catastrophic events.

Admittedly, there is debate about what tests to run. And quite often the results look like hieroglyphics. It's a confusing and sometimes overwhelming topic to the layperson. To cut through this, we encourage you to find the right guide to help navigate these intimidating areas. A trusted physician can help you translate your lab values into usable information, and with the right information, you can make the proper adjustments to live a longer, healthier life.

"When we prioritize our thoughts and emotions, the things that are important to us and the things we are willing to give up move to the forefront of our thoughts and actions."
–Notes from the Doc

In addition to being free from injury and illness, we want to face our days with vitality and capacity. Let's start by asking ourselves, "How do I feel today?" Be sure to assess your physical state as well as your emotions. This is where the RedeFit Model comes into play and is beneficial in helping you feel better. For example, if we don't have strong relationships in our life, we won't have a sense of belonging. This may make us feel disconnected or even depressed. Also, if we are overwhelmed by all the little things in life and not having any fun, then we won't feel good.

On the other hand, if we set our sights too high, like trying to eat perfectly and fail, we will feel bad about not meeting our goals. And we will feel like a failure. With the RedeFit approach, we simplify the areas you are working on and recommend small incremental changes. That way you can set achievable goals and make progress toward those goals, feeling a sense of accomplishment along the way. The same goes for the physical side of the RedeFit Model. If you are weak, winded easily, or so tight it's hard to move, you won't feel good. With our approach, we help you make strides every day, which will make you feel better.

How your mind and body feel right now is your first gauge of health. Our actions leading up to this moment will determine how we feel today. Improving your health is challenging because it's not a quick fix. But don't worry. Even if we don't feel good right now, we can change that with the right plan. This will take some time—one workout, one meal, one day might not be the tipping point for us to feel great, but it's a step in the right direction. With each thing you do that supports your health and well-being, you contribute to feeling good about your accomplishments. It's important to remember we only have control over the present moment. What's been done in the past is history, and what you need to do in the future has not yet arrived. Your focus should be on what you can do right now.

Health is a broad and multifaceted topic. Although all the categories are important, two parts of the RedeFit Model are critical in supporting and optimizing health—stress management and nutrition. Both have a dramatic impact on your health.

Defining proper nutrition is covered in detail in Chapter 8 and gives you a breakdown of approaches for promoting nutrition. Nutrition is a foundational pillar of health. It is not possible to eat consistently unhealthily and be healthy. We define unhealthy food as high in calories but low in nutrients. This seems very straightforward, but most people we work with are trying to be healthy while still eating unhealthily. This mindset is associated with short-term reward vs. long-term goals. The short-term reward is eating something right now just because it tastes good, not because it is health-promoting. If we want to promote health, we need food that is nutrient-dense. Side note: it can also taste good. This is the key: to find foods you like that are also nutrient-dense. Remember the two are not mutually exclusive.

The beauty of eating healthily is that it is becoming more popular, and with popularity comes more options. You can search online for a healthy version of your favorite food and find some amazing substitutes that will lower the calories of the meal and add more nutrients. A few examples include spaghetti squash substituted for regular noodles, infused oil and balsamic as a replacement for high-fat salad dressing, and fruit-infused sparkling water or kombucha instead of soda. Another way to support healthy eating is by changing your environment. For example, cooking at home as opposed to eating out, or hosting guests at your house instead of going to their homes. That way you have control over the food and drinks you serve and eat.

Stress management is another foundational tool of health and is covered in detail in Chapter 5. It must be addressed for optimal health. With an increased ability to manage stress, your mind and body will be able to relax and recover at a more efficient rate which will promote long-term health.

"Meditating or thinking about your goals for five minutes a day is an amazing way to reduce stress." –Notes from the Doc

----

When you are stressed, your ability to digest and absorb food decreases. We discussed the importance of a healthy diet. Now we need to make sure your body is supported in doing its job and utilizing the nutrients those foods provide. When your body is stressed, blood flow to your digestive system can be limited, resulting in constipation, or food moving too quickly through your body. You will feel uncomfortable and your body won't maximize proper absorption of the nutrients.

We cover stress management in more depth in Chapter 5, but

let's also look at stress management here. Begin by asking yourself, "What am I doing today that my future self will thank me for?" Identifying and making small adjustments to your environment and life can support you in eating healthily on a regular basis, managing your stress, and engaging in daily physical activity. Your future self will thank you for these modifications. You'll quickly be feeling healthier and be moving toward a future, and your lab testing outcomes will reflect this.

Let's look at some exceptions not consistent with our guidelines. Does this sound familiar? *Did you hear about the guy who smoked, drank, ate whatever he wanted and lived to be over 100? How about this one? Did you hear about the guy who worked out all the time, ate nothing but healthy food, and died of a heart attack at the age of 40?*

There are two misconceptions here. First, it seems a lot of people have heard about "these guys" but very few actually know one of these guys. Second, there is always an exception to the rule. Some people are so genetically gifted their body filters out all their poor health choices and optimizes the good. On the other hand, some are genetically predisposed in a way that no matter what they do they will have a shorter than average lifespan. For both the genetically gifted and those people genetically disposed to certain health conditions, addressing the categories of the RedeFit Model can still have a major impact on their quality of life. The way our parents and grandparents ate and the environment we live in play a major role in our health. By taking the time to examine some of the key markers with regular testing, we have more details to make informed decisions about our future health.

DON'T BE FOOLED

Health isn't as sexy as six-pack abs. It's not as marketable as losing weight quickly and becoming slender and lean. Health doesn't make for a great social media post like someone triumphantly crossing the finish line of their first marathon. Even so, you'll be hard-pressed to find a factor that plays a greater role in your experience and engagement with life. Health is the very platform that your life depends on. It is your foundation for living a full and meaningful life.

The table below presents recommendations for improving your health. In the ADD column, we propose behaviors to add to your daily activities. In the LIMIT column, we include behaviors to limit in your daily activities.

ADD
Include daily movement.
Schedule a doctor's visit/yearly check-up.
Invest in a fitness professional.
LIMIT
Reduce the amount of time you're sitting throughout the day.
Avoid mindless late-night snacking.
Limit alcohol intake.

For a deeper understanding of these and other strategies, visit TheRedefit.com

NOTES FROM THE DOC

Why do people with good blood pressure regularly monitor it using drug store blood pressure cuffs? Why are we so willing to jump on the scale when we are content with our weight, but we avoid it like the plague most other days? There are many facets to who we are and why we do things, but the above examples and the others you may have imagined are often due to our almost insatiable need for instant gratification. Modern devices and our corresponding culture are full of opportunities for instant gratification. If we feel lonely, we jump on social media for social interactions, even if they're only virtual. If we want or need something, we order it today and receive it tomorrow.

Why are we so attracted to instant gratification, and what does this have to do with health? Instant gratification is most often associated with what the famed psychologist, Sigmund Freud, labeled the "pleasure principle." This term represented our basic self—much like children—our desire to have our needs met immediately and avoid pain or discomfort—even that which comes from waiting for something. As such, by default, in Freudian psychoanalysis, adulthood was defined by the ability to delay gratification for a larger, long-term pursuit. Yet pursuing some forms of immediate gratification as adults can be essential to relieving stress and experiencing what our diverse and rich environments offer. This balancing act of instant vs. delayed gratification is complex at best.

So, how do we know if instant gratification is bad or when the balance with delayed gratification is out of whack? A great measure of this has to do with our goals or lack of them. Goal setting is highly correlated with delayed gratification and overall success.

In other words, if a goal is set to run a marathon, start a business, have a family, and so on, the behaviors necessary to achieve those goals become clear. If you are really excited about completing a marathon, you might more easily skip a night out with friends to make sure you can successfully stick with your training plan the next morning. If you want to start a business, it becomes evident that saving money or taking time away from your favorite TV show to work on the business plan is the right choice. The issue most of us face is that when we delay gratification we can often feel temporarily dissatisfied, especially because there are no guarantees in life that the goals we set, and work toward will ever happen. So, why would we want to go through the discomfort, even pain, of delayed gratification?

In 1960 Stanford researchers conducted a now popular study to investigate whether delay gratification pays off. They provided children with a choice: they could have one marshmallow immediately or wait 15 minutes and have two. While the children waited and contemplated their decision, they were left alone with the first marshmallow; they could functionally cave in at any time, even if they were hoping to wait for the second marshmallow. The children that were able to delay gratification to receive two marshmallows, were subsequently—decades later—evaluated to be less likely to have behavior issues, scored better on standardized tests, and had better health than their immediate gratification counterparts. Subsequent research continues to point to the clear health benefits of delayed gratification.

The importance of delayed gratification affects health in many ways, both mentally and physically. From a mental standpoint, the difference is really pleasure vs. happiness. Few adults will argue that things like sex and drugs provide pleasure, typically in a more instant gratification framework. However, they are not synonymous with happiness, often quite the opposite. Ironically, when the instant gratification has passed, and we are not happy, we repeat the behaviors to provide temporary relief from our reality. As such, this feedback loop creates an ongoing destructive cycle. When we do this with our nutrition and our stress-coping responses, we are amplifying our physical challenges. Over-eating, eating foods that are nutritionally void and calorically dense, skipping workouts, or doing one more thing for one more person become escape mechanisms from the realities that are in our control. These are examples of ways in which we struggle with balance. In the literature, this is often referred to as a lack of self-control or willpower. I am often asked how to enhance these qualities. There is no magic pill for more self-control or willpower. There is no immediate way to increase the ability to have delayed gratification. As frustrating as that is, the reality is that more often than not, we actually have the willpower; we simply have not harnessed it.

Think about something over which you have self-control or willpower. Remember the time you declined a fun evening out with friends because someone you cared about needed something? What about the sacrifice you made at work to help the team meet a deadline? Or when you bit your tongue when "that uncle" said something you disagreed with, so you could keep peace at the dinner table. Our willpower often is tied to the values and goals we hold. When we prioritize our thoughts and emotions, the things that are important to us and the things we are willing to give up move to the forefront of our thoughts and actions.

Take a moment to think about this question. What does your health mean to you?

- Time with people you care about?
- Opportunities to see new places and meet new people?
- Extended opportunities to make an impact and serve society?
- Time and energy to achieve personal and professional goals?

As I mentioned at the outset, the relationship for us between having our needs and wants met immediately and being playful is a complicated balance. If it wasn't, we wouldn't struggle with health issues. So, we need to identify ways to keep the balance, such as goal setting and using our modern devices. For the first time in history, we have high-tech tools at our disposal to help us maintain this balance.

How should you begin? First, set your intention. What do you want to get from your health? It can be any of the above examples or a host of others. Then as you decline dessert, prioritize sleep over excessive drinking, and exercise, you realize you are not depriving yourself of pleasure; you are securing your happiness and moving toward your goals. Second, use tools to help you track your progress and to provide instant gratification. If you have never tracked your sleep or food, an app that reminds you to log in and then celebrates winning streaks can be a powerful way to get pleasure from your successes no matter how small. Meditating or thinking about your goals for five minutes a day is an amazing way to reduce stress. Use technology to guide you through and to celebrate with others, allowing instant gratification to be part of the equation. Just commit to finding people, such as doctors and coaches, and tools, like apps and other technology, to help you plan and reward yourself along the way.

Chapter 10
Physical

The three elements of the physical side—stamina, flexibility, and strength—must be in balance to live your life to the fullest.

When it comes to the physical aspects of the RedeFit Model—strength, flexibility, and stamina—there's no doubt that a healthier body equals an improved quality of life. A healthier cardiovascular system supports an active lifestyle—everything from evening walks to playing with the children to riding your bike or playing a game of tennis. An improved range of motion translates into easier movement and a sense of freedom. Extra strength is helpful when opening a stuck pickle jar lid and avoiding falls. The benefits of training for a healthier body are undeniable. We can imagine the freedom and happiness that would accompany it. Then why do so many of us lack the healthy, lean, capable body we desire? What's stopping us? There are two major hurdles we encounter when pursuing our optimal physical health: failing to launch and doubling down on our current approach. Let's explore both.

"Why do so many of us have failure-to-launch syndrome when consistently engaging in activities that promote health and fitness? Because we are hard-wired to preserve energy."
–Notes from the Doc

FAILING TO LAUNCH

Very often the initial hurdle is not knowing where to start. There is so much fitness information available that defining a starting point is a herculean task. After we pick one, doubt quickly creeps in. *Is this the right program for me? How do I make progress? How do I know if it's working? Is this too much or should I be doing more? Is the newly unveiled program better than the one I'm currently considering?* The questions multiply, and we soon feel overwhelmed. This place of doubt and uncertainty is not a strong foundation from which to build a new habit.

With the thousands of fitness options, it's easy to see why many of us default to the path of least resistance—to do nothing. The thought is: *Better to save our time and energy than waste it on an approach we're unsure of.* After all, our time is limited and valuable, our energy already rationed out to the many roles we must fulfill. It's not surprising that so few raise the sail and launch.

If being physically active is new to you, that's okay. You're not alone. The RedeFit approach is designed for your success. We understand that your time and energy are valuable, and we want you to use them as efficiently as possible to get and maintain the results you want. We are your guides in navigating your unique journey to your goals. You can feel confident that you're in good hands.

"Behavior that is maintained is typically reinforced by internal or external rewards." –Notes from the Doc

----

DOUBLING DOWN

Let's say you're one of the few who have chosen a fitness path and embarked on it. Chances are good that you enjoy one part of the physical piece more than the others. Maybe you gravitate toward resistance training to the detriment of your flexibility or stamina. Or perhaps you regularly attend yoga classes and neglect your stamina and strength. Maybe you're a cardio warrior who puts countless miles on your feet but never touches a weight nor works on flexibility. If you find yourself identifying with any of these approaches, you should know this is extremely common. We often default to the area about which we feel the most competent and confident. When we find it, we go all in. And, although energy and enthusiasm toward a fitness goal are commendable, a problem soon arises with this approach. You probably know already because you've experienced the shortcomings of this approach. It results in a body that is out of balance.

When you began, you gravitated toward strength, stamina, or flexibility. Initially, you likely saw quick, noticeable results. But when the beginner's progress soon wore off, you doubled down on your efforts to continue making progress. You invested extra time, miles, or reps. This approach worked in the short run, but all too soon your results plateaued. This sequence of events can be quite frustrating. Putting all our eggs in one basket leads to stagnation, predisposition for injury, and lack of overall capacity.

We must maintain a balance between strength, stamina, and flexibility. We'll explore that balance later in this chapter.

The three elements of the physical side must be in balance to live your life to the fullest. The only exception would be for someone competing at a very high level. The importance of achieving balance and competency in all areas comes down to your ability to perform daily functions and participate in activities that you love at your optimal level. Are you strong enough to pick up the small children in your life—your nieces, nephews, and grandchildren? Can you walk up two flights of stairs without becoming winded? Are you able to reach in the back seat of your car without hurting your shoulder? Are you able to play a pickup game of the sport you once enjoyed? Having strength, flexibility, and stamina will help you live a lean, healthy, and happy life.

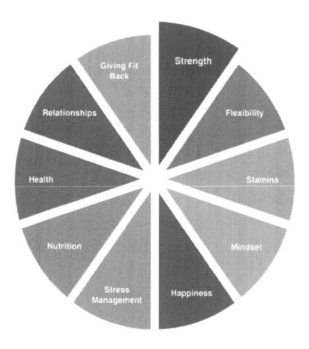

STRENGTH

Why is strength important? Strength is one of the best indicators for longevity. Maintaining your strength will enable you to keep doing the activities you love, and it will help protect your body from day-to-day damage. When we discuss strength, we are not referring to the extremes. We are not advocating competing in a lifting competition, doing crazy workouts, or going to the gym every day. What we want for you is what you want—to perform movements on a consistent basis that will make you stronger and move better.

When thinking about strengthening your body, think about it like the RedeFit Model. Balance is key. We have all seen people who don't strike this balance. For example, some people will inappropriately incorporate strength training, focusing on just one part of their body or only on exercises they are good at. A perfect example is guys who do only arm and chest workouts. Admittedly, they become much stronger in these areas, but this singular focus can lead to injuries or dysfunction. You'll see our strength training examples; our focus is on the entire body—on creating and maintaining balanced function.

When starting your new strength training program, it is important to consider both past and present injuries. Step one is to always consult your doctor before beginning any exercise or training routine. Step two is to slowly get into a program and don't overdo it. Begin very conservatively and slowly ramp up volume and intensity. For example, take a past knee injury. The leg that suffered the injury typically becomes weaker either due to surgery or from compensation away from that leg to avoid pain. In this situation, it is important to focus more on unilateral work vs. bilateral work.

This means performing movements that focus on one leg at a time, like a step-up instead of movements that work both legs at a time, like a squat. With a careful approach like this, start with the weaker side and mirror the same volume and intensity on the stronger side. Eventually, they will get much closer in strength. You'll find numerous unilateral exercises in the RedeFit Model to help navigate situations like this.

One of the beauties of strength training is that if a given movement causes you pain or if you just don't like it, skip it. There are plenty of alternatives. For example, if you have always hated push-ups, then don't do them. Instead, you could do an incline dumbbell press, tricep extension, flat barbell bench press, or high plank hold. The secret is finding a program you can stick with and identifying movements you enjoy.

Strength training can be done with any form of resistance, like weights, bands, cables, machines or even your body alone. For most people, starting with just your body weight is a great way to begin. Start slowly and easily. Then over time, add more resistance and make the strength training more complex if needed. Too often with strength training, people do too much too soon. This can lead to excessive soreness or even injury. Remember our maxim: consistency over intensity. We are on this journey for life, not a few weeks.

If strength is your number one priority from your assessment, try to complete three strength training sessions per week. Then on the other four days, choose activities you enjoy. This could include flexibility and/or cardio sessions from the RedeFit Model or something as simple as a walk. It's okay if you miss a day. Our aim is to move every day. If you don't have time for a complete session on a given day, no worries. Devote the time you do have to movement—something as simple as a short walk or a portion of a training session. Make sure to keep the habit alive. Put your training in your planner, make it a priority, and do your best to stick to it.

At Home Strength Workout Examples

Choose an exercise from each category.

Lower Body Push	Upper Body Push	Lower Body Pull	Upper Body Pull	Core
Squat	Pushup	Stability ball leg curl	Band pull apart	Tuck hold
Stationary lunge	Kneeling pushup	Dumbbell straight leg deadlift	Bandpull-down	Tuck up
Step up	Dumbbell lateral raise	Bridge	Bent over dumbbell row	Plank
Walking lunge	Dumbbell shoulder press	Elevated bridge	Bent over dumbbell lateral raise	Arch hold

Aim to complete 12-15 reps of that exercise in 40 seconds, then take 20 seconds break and then proceed to the next exercise. Repeat that process until you've completed all 5 exercise categories. Rest as needed after that round. Build up your capacity and eventually aim to complete 4-6 rounds.

For a deeper understanding of these and other strategies, visit TheRedefit.com

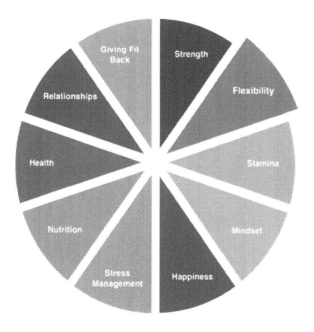

FLEXIBILITY

Why is flexibility important? In our discussion about strength, we stressed the importance of remaining strong through a full range of motion. If we are so tight, we can't straighten our arms or squat, then how can we strengthen that area? We can't. Flexibility will give us the ability to strengthen through a full range of motion, enable us to move without pain, and make everyday tasks much easier. When we lack flexibility, our body will compensate in other joints to cope with the diminished range of motion. This compensation can lead to discomfort and pain. The appropriate amount of flexibility not only allows us to gain strength but can be preventative in avoiding pain. Your suitable range of motion will be unique to you. We don't expect you to perform in the Cirque du Soleil, become a gymnast, or even practice yoga every day. Flexibility is not about extremes; it is about practicing movements on a consistent basis that will give you a greater range of motion and ease of movement.

The great thing about flexibility training is that it can be done anywhere and anytime. By working in some stretching throughout your day, you will feel better and counteract much of the poor posture that day-to-day activities reinforce. Sitting at a desk, driving a car, and looking at our cell phone encourage bad habits, such as a forward-leaning head, craned neck, rounded shoulders and back, and tight hip flexors, which can lead to pain and increase your chances of injury. The RedeFit Model offers daily movements for countering this position, so you can maintain proper posture and a full range of motion.

Many people who hope to improve flexibility try a yoga class. This can be a very effective way to improve your flexibility, but just be aware that referring to "yoga" is a lot like saying "working out." There's no one size fits all. In fact, there are many different styles from very relaxing to very intense. And the style and intensity of a yoga class typically depend on the teacher. Yoga terminology and the students' level can be intimidating if you're in a class that's too advanced. Don't let this scare you away. Just be aware that classes vary greatly, and if you're new to the practice, you might benefit from finding a class for beginners.

To increase flexibility, it's important to combine stretching, positioning, and breathing. Stretching in the right position can enhance movement. A common example is when you stand with your chest and butt extended, also known as an anterior pelvic tilt. This tilt tightens the hamstrings, so just by adjusting that position—tilting the pelvis inward—before stretching your hamstrings, you will increase its effectiveness. Deep relaxing breaths also facilitate stretching and flexibility. Your body has a built-in protective mechanism against injury, so when you stretch in a position you're not used to, your body will tense up. Deep relaxing breaths will signal to your body that it's not in trouble and allow you to further your movement.

If flexibility is your number one priority from your assessment, complete three flexibility sessions per week. On the other four days, add activities you enjoy, such as strength or cardio sessions from the RedeFit approach. It's okay to miss a day. Our aim is to incorporate flexibility training or movement every day. Perhaps you don't have time for a complete session on a given day. That's okay.

Use the time you do have to keep some movement or flexibility training in your day. This could include something as simple as a short stretch through your favorite movement or completing just part of a flexibility session. It doesn't need to be complicated. Make sure to keep the habit alive. Put your flexibility training in your planner, make it a priority, and do your best to stick to it.

For a deeper understanding of these and other strategies, visit TheRedefit.com.

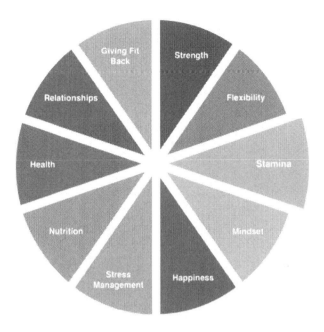

STAMINA

Why is stamina so important? Stamina gives us the ability to do things longer, whether it's playing with our children, competing in a game of tennis, or simply climbing stairs without becoming winded. You can increase your stamina in many different ways— by doing higher reps with weights or by running, biking, and swimming. The key benefit is being able to do more of what you love without getting tired or winded.

We encourage you to approach stamina like strength and flexibility—avoid the extremes. We are not advocating that you run an ultramarathon, compete in a triathlon, or spend countless hours on the road every day. Instead, we encourage you to move consistently in a way basis that will increase your stamina and improve your ease of movement.

Stamina-based workouts can be completed in your living room with your body weight alone, around your neighborhood, on a trail, or in a conditioning class. You can even use weights to improve stamina. While lower reps and heavier weights are the emphasis for strength training, lower weights and increased reps are the focus for building stamina. This simple change shifts the emphasis from strength training to stamina. For example, squatting while lifting weights can help you achieve either goal. Using heavier weights while doing fewer reps translates into strength training, whereas lifting lighter weights while doing higher reps facilitates stamina training. Which one is better? It depends on your goals. If your physical score identified strength as your number one priority, add more weight and decrease your reps. If your physical score indicated that stamina was your number one priority, decrease the weight and increase the reps. Both are important in maintaining a good quality of life, but the one that is more important at this moment depends on your assessment.

Stamina is another great example of how fitness is unique to the individual. If you get winded walking from your car to the store, then strolling around your block is your first step. If you train regularly but just focus on one of the other two areas on the physical side of the wheel, then maybe a light jog, a long swim, or a long bike ride might be a better option. The secret is doing something a little harder than what you already can do. Remember you're not training to win a race; you are working to improve your stamina in an enjoyable way.

To build consistency with stamina training, find an activity you enjoy. Take running for example. If our clients hate running, we don't ask them to do it. But if they love running, we urge them to do what they enjoy. There are many ways to improve stamina that don't include running. You can swim, bike, or lift weights at higher reps to name a few. If you enjoy the activity, you will be consistent, and your consistency will produce progress in your stamina. And, as you progress, you can incrementally increase the challenge and variation you bring to your stamina training.

If stamina is your number one priority from your assessment, complete three stamina sessions per week. On the other four days, choose something enjoyable, which could include flexibility or strength sessions from the RedeFit Model. If you miss a day, it's not a problem. Our aim is to encourage you to move every day. It's fine if you don't have time for a complete stamina session on a given day. Use the time you have to keep some movement in your day. This could include something as simple as a short walk or completing just part of one of your training sessions. Make sure to keep the habit alive. Put your training in your planner, make it a priority, and do your best to stick to it.

STAMINA EXAMPLES

Stamina can be divided into two categories: 1) Steady-state and 2) Intervals. It is important to address both. Address either steady state or intervals on your stamina training days and then rotate to the other option on your next stamina training day. If you are in the beginning stage, use your stamina days to walk 7000 steps. After you are consistently doing that, graduate to the novice level.

Below is a progression of how you could address your stamina training. Start conservatively and select a level you can confidently complete. Remember, our mantra is consistency over intensity. We can always do more tomorrow but can't undo our soreness if we do too much today. After you're consistently completing the stage you're on, advance to the next level.

1. Steady State Cardio
- Beginner: 7k steps/day
- Novice: run/walk 1 mile
- Intermediate: run/walk 2 miles
- Advanced: run/walk 3 miles
- Very Advanced: run/walk 4 miles

2. Intervals
- Beginner: no intervals, focus on 7k steps per day
- Novice: a work-to-rest ratio of 1:4 for 4-8 rounds
- Example: 30 seconds of work, 120-second break repeated 4-8 times
- Intermediate 1: a work-to-rest ratio of 1:3 for 5-10 rounds
- Example: 30 seconds of work, 90-second break repeated 5-10 times
- Intermediate 2: a work-to-rest ratio of 1:2 for 5-10 rounds
- Example: 30 seconds of work, 60-second break repeated 5-10 times
- Advanced: a work-to-rest ratio of 1:1 for 6 to 12 rounds
- Example: 30 seconds of work, 30-second break repeated 6 to 12 times
- Very Advanced: a work-to-rest ratio of 2:1 for 8-14 rounds
- Example: 40 seconds of work, 20-second break repeated 8-14 times

3. Possible Movements for Intervals

- Walk
- Run
- Swim
- Row
- Bike
- Elliptical
- Jump rope
- Body weight exercises: squat, lunge, jump, etc.

The table below presents recommendations for improving your physical health and fitness. In the ADD column, we propose behaviors to add to your daily activities. In the LIMIT column, we include behaviors to limit in your daily activities.

ADD
Ensure you incorporate some physical activity into your routine this week.
Mix up the activities you do—try something new.
Find someone to do your activities with.
LIMIT
Avoid days with no physical activity.
Minimize prolonged periods of sedentary activity.
Refrain from too much screen time.

For a deeper understanding of these and other strategies, visit TheRedefit.com.

NOTES FROM THE DOC

This chapter is about the importance of movement and activity. Since grade school and the advent of the physical education class, this truth has been an often-heard refrain. Then why is it that many of us have failure-to-launch syndrome when consistently engaging in activities that promote health and fitness? Would you believe it's in large part because we are hard-wired to preserve our energy? Think about it. Until the industrial revolution, humans were required to functionally kill and grow our food for basic survival. This lifestyle was so energy intensive, our predecessors became very adept at preserving energy when it was not required for survival.

Fast forward to today's lifestyle. The ease by which modern humans acquire food, especially fats and carbs, far outweighs our minimal daily energy expenditures for survival. In turn, we as a society are experiencing an increased number of unique health issues. Just by reading this book in an effort to impact your overall health, you understand this. You are unique. You recognize that to fully benefit from present-day opportunities for a prosperous life, key lifestyle changes are needed to override our preservation tendencies. We *need* to move.

Our tendency to preserve happens daily in many ways. When you choose to sit versus stand, take the escalator instead of the stairs, or hit the snooze button rather than getting out of bed to go work out, your body is simply defaulting to energy-saving mode. However, another aspect of our modern world is that we have many more opportunities to explore and enjoy activities and experiences that do not involve survival. We can travel and spend more quality time with the people we value. We have much more time to devote to these things as our life expectancy has more than doubled from our Stone Age ancestors. As such, it no longer makes sense to lie around preserving energy when we can go to the park with the little ones in our lives or seek new adventures, big and small. Finally, and perhaps most notable, we have the opportunity, more than any other time in our history, to positively impact others with our resources, talents, and energy.

LAUNCHING

In the sections on strength, flexibility, and endurance, we recommended movements and activities to get started on your journey to improved physical health. We anticipate that you will find one or more of these a good fit for your current lifestyle and goals. Yet how do we get past our failure-to-launch tendencies and also maintain our new behaviors? The first step is to fully understand what this means. How many times have you seen an exercise product ad touting how fast and easy it is to use? All the time—right? My personal favorites are those that show a beautiful couple in a mansion with a killer view working out together. They finish their workout looking perfectly put together and then enjoy an elaborate sit-down breakfast with their family. The children miraculously come down right when they are finished in a good mood with no needs. How often does that happen? Never. The reality is that for most of us it takes UPS-level logistics to coordinate our days, family, and work to maintain a consistent level of activity. Yet, that is okay, because that is the point. The point is not to do it perfectly under all conditions. Just like anything else in our lives: if we value it, we figure it out.

The goal is not to make hard things easier; the goal is to make the hard things automatic.

Don't get me wrong, finding fun and engaging ways to keep our bodies healthy for all the activities is encouraged. But if the path of least resistance was the secret, there would be no need for the RedeFit Model because everyone would have this figured out. Once we acknowledge and embrace that this will take some effort, the next step is to create new and modify old habits that support consistency over intensity.

Easy is not part of why you do the work, but desire is.

The foundation for developing any new habit is desire. You literally must want a new habit. New Year's resolutions are a great example. How many times have you or someone you knew set a New Year resolution and then broke it within the first few hours or days? This is really not about willpower; it is about desire. A new habit needs to be something you actually want, not something you feel pressured into working toward. Think about when you work very hard at something. It's typically because you truly want something (internal satisfaction, paycheck) or value it (family, community service). Easy is not part of why you do the work, but desire is.

Once you have acknowledged the rationale for the hard work, it's important to do a little up-front work to set yourself up for success.

1. *Habit replacement*: Instead of adding something else to your life, this is about creating opportunities to build the time and opportunities into your already packed lifestyle. Do you tend to unwind at night with the TV? Great, no judgment here. The increasing array of options offers some amazing opportunities to learn and experience many new things (think: Travel Channel). Let's say you put in about 90 minutes of TV a night on average. Can you take a 15-minute break for movement? Or during each commercial, challenge yourself to some push-ups or sit-ups. Many of the options we recommended under strength and flexibility would work great. When waiting on a child's extramural practice, can you walk with another parent while you catch up? Or perhaps take one flight of stairs when leaving work. Again, we are not adding time; we are replacing energy-conserving habits with those that support your new goal and lifestyle.

2. *Get in touch with your emotions:* This strategy has firm roots in cognitive behavior change and is effective in addressing the procrastination and avoidance tendencies we all have. Write down on a whiteboard, a pad of paper, or the refrigerator the behaviors you want to incorporate into your life. For example, let's say you would like to move for 30 minutes a day. Then, each day, mark whether you accomplished this goal and the emotion you feel about it. Be honest with yourself. If you did it, and feel great about it, think about that and express that positive emotion to yourself and others. By doing this you are pairing positive emotions with the hard work and the effort you put forth. Over time your brain starts to look at the goal to get that positive feeling—much like comfort food does for many people. Similarly, if you didn't manage to get

that activity in and feel regret, embarrassment, or disappointment, connect with that emotion. This pairs the inactivity with feelings you are not interested in repeating. This cues your brain that inactivity does not feel great. These are all powerful cues for the brain to engage in new behaviors. The point here is not to beat yourself up or gloat to yourself and friends. Rather, it is to create cognitive and emotional wins for yourself to move the momentum in the desired direction. This is also why it's so important not to set unreasonable goals, start small, get those wins, and then work up. Then the hard stuff becomes achievable and rewarding.

3. *Make adjustments to your environment:* A significant amount of behavior research has demonstrated that our behavior is driven by specific cues, many learned from the way we live. What environmental cues are associated with the habits you want to change? Do your feet hurt every time you have tried to walk or run? Those shoes will signal pain and discomfort each time you think about putting them on for a walk. Go see an athletic shoe specialist (many running stores have in-house specialists) and make sure you are fitted for the right shoe.

Do you revel in finding the best parking spot at the mall or work? Can you instead challenge yourself to find the spot farthest away, so you can get your steps in? Is the remote control close to your favorite TV chair? Keep it in another room. Next time you do laundry, dump all the clean clothes on that chair. Then fold them before you sit down. Where do you keep your gym bag? Is it in an easy-to-access location and packed the night before? If you do your movement at home before the day starts, can you pack your briefcase and lunches the night before to ensure you have uninterrupted time in the morning? Create cues that promote the modified habits you want to establish. They will signify to your brain to act and will create less lifestyle tension around accomplishing them.

4. Create a reinforcement for yourself: Lots of fitness programs come with handy apps and charts to track your progress. It's important to celebrate the wins and see change, both large and small. However, if you are not a numbers or charting type of person, this may not excite you. Be planful about how you encourage yourself and fuel your sense of fulfillment. If you like quality time, who can you plan this with?

Lately, I have been working on learning handstands. For many reasons, this does not come naturally to me. It's tough and some days are filled with frustration. However, as my youngest is about to leave for college, precious time with him is even more of a priority for me. He likes the challenges of doing handstands, so we go to class and practice together. Of course, he is picking it up so much faster than me!

If you are someone who feels appreciated and cared for through tangible gifts, or if you like to shop, tap into that preference. First, create your movement/activity goal and then for your first small win or several big wins (depending on if you want more small things or a few bigger ones) buy a new accessory or clothing item to enhance your workout experience. When I first started running seriously, I was a graduate student with no disposable income. I wanted to work out and running was the cheapest option because it only required me and some sidewalks. I had very inexpensive sneakers not designed for long-term running. I wanted to make sure I launched this new habit in earnest before I invested my grocery money into new shoes. So, I set a goal to run an average of three days across several weeks. Once I hit that goal, I rewarded myself with new running shoes. This set me on an awesome 20-year running experience. You do not have to wait to hit a major goal over a long period of time. You can reinforce yourself for taking the first step with something smaller, such as a free app that tracks your heart rate, or a new water bottle. Behavior that is maintained is typically reinforced by internal or external rewards. What reinforces your behavior may often evolve as the behavior evolves. Whatever you decide to do, take the time to celebrate your effort in ways that are meaningful to you.

Chapter 11
Giving Fit Back (GFB)

"The best asset we have for making a contribution to the world is ourselves. If we underinvest in ourselves, and by that, I mean our minds, our bodies, and our spirits, we damage the very tool we need to make our highest contribution." –Greg McKeown

----

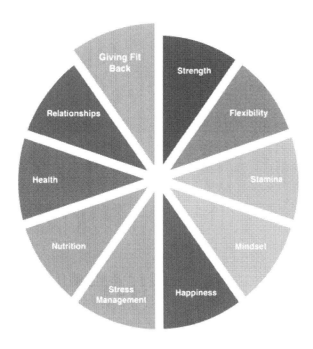

Why is "Giving Fit Back" the last chapter in our book? Whether intentional or unintentional, your actions influence those around you. Every action has gravity—it pulls on the behaviors of the people in your life. The way you behave influences every aspect of their lives—the words used with your children, the activities you pursue, your physical activity or lack thereof, and the food you eat. Through your actions, your tribes receive subtle cues about acceptable and unacceptable behavior. By becoming leaner, healthier, and happier, you can influence and inspire the people around you to do the same.

To have the greatest impact, we encourage you to start with you. You are your greatest asset in positively influencing your world. With the other categories of fitness in working order, you're in an optimal position to begin intentionally improving the lives of the people in your tribes.

"Lighthouses don't go running all over an island looking for boats to save; they just stand there shining." –Anne Lamott

----

The best way to influence is by being a lighthouse for others. Of course, you will influence the people around you from the outset of this program, but you must work on yourself before working with others. We can't underscore this point enough. And keep in mind: the most important part of being a fitness influencer is living the fit lifestyle—being a stellar example for those around you.

Your journey to this point has undoubtedly had its challenges, but they're ones you have overcome. Now you'll face a new challenge. Once your fitness is in balance, it is one of the hardest obstacles you will face. What's the challenge? Seeing the people closest to you unwilling to make the changes that would lead them to greater well-being. Don't try to convince them or judge them if they resist a fit lifestyle. It's your job to live a healthy life, set an example, and be there for guidance when the time is right. You are their lighthouse—illuminating their path and showing them the way.

GFB TO YOUR FAMILY

Family members can be simultaneously the easiest and hardest people in your life to which to give fit back. They are the easiest because of your close contact and relationships. They are the hardest because you were born into your family; you didn't choose them based on common values. If you're fortunate, your family members share similar values, but this isn't always the case. You likely don't love them any less for having a different world view, although sometimes tensions arise within families over political, religious, or other differences in values.

When family members see you living a better life, they will take notice. Leading by example is much more powerful than trying to persuade them to make healthier choices. In fact, sometimes preaching to the unconverted can make family members more resistant and less likely to come around. For example, how has it worked to urge loved ones who don't love veggies to eat more? As the saying goes, the proof is in the pudding. When they see a leaner, healthier, happier you, they will be inspired to follow suit.

For many reading this book, you're part of a generation sandwiched between two family obligations—the challenge of raising children *and* taking care of aging parents. Both have their unique opportunities and obstacles.

Children offer a unique opportunity to give fit back. Besides providing for their basic needs, being a positive fitness influencer may be one of the most important jobs you have as their parent, teacher, and mentor. While they are under your care, your influence is immense. Children's early interactions and examples can steer them to a lifetime of health and happiness or lead them astray.

Again, this comes from you first. There is real power in being a living example of lean, healthy, and happy. It is unconvincing to resort to: "Do as I say, not as I do." Children see through the words and mimic the behaviors they observe, which is why it's important to be the embodiment of healthy behaviors and then reinforce those behaviors with your words.

Positively influencing your children makes your home life much more enjoyable. If your children aren't healthy, your life is far more challenging. Doing what you can to facilitate their health and happiness can remove some of the avoidable stress and challenges. Also, having your children on board helps you maintain your happy, healthy life. We have had many clients who eat unhealthily by finishing their children's plates of French fries or chicken nuggets or catering to their demands for sugary snacks in the pantry. The unique opportunity that exists with young children is that you can control aspects of their environment, such as the easily accessible foods. You can set up the environment for success for them and for you.

You also have an obligation to your elders—your parents and grandparents. They can be difficult because they've seen the pendulum in the fitness and nutrition worlds swing from one extreme to the other and back again. They have also witnessed the fitness boom replete with gadgets, equipment, extreme diets, and bad tasting "healthy food." Here are just a few examples of things we've heard from our parents.

"Eggs are bad for you, then they are good, now they are bad again. Nobody knows."

"The worse it tastes, the better it is for you."

"It doesn't matter; it all causes cancer."

It is also difficult because our parents lived in a very different time. When speaking with people your parents' and grandparents' age, you'll hear stories that sound so foreign, like splitting a soda with a sibling once a week or getting an orange for Christmas. Just a generation or two ago, a soda was a special treat. Now it has become the norm and extremely abundant. How would a child today react if they only got an orange for Christmas? Previous generations come from a time in which people worked hard, didn't worry about macros or calories, and were rewarded with food and treats. Because they view the world differently, they need a different strategy to elicit change.

A key to working with parents is making small changes and letting them experience the results. Another strategy is for them to hear the same good advice you're delivering but from another source. It can be tough to take advice from someone whose diaper they used to change. Partnering them with a fitness professional who is on the same page as you or a trusted doctor who can deliver smart real-world strategies can sidestep the "I changed your diaper" objection and steer them toward better health.

GFB TO YOUR FRIENDS

The beauty of friends is that you get to pick them. If you enjoy their company and they don't negatively affect your overall fitness, it doesn't matter how they live. If you're a pleaser, though, it will be difficult not to be influenced. For example, if your group of friends enjoys happy hour, has too much wine with dinner, and binge-watches Netflix on the weekends, it will be a challenge for you to spend time with them and not partake. But if, on the other hand, your friends sample the new kombucha on tap Friday night, go for hikes on Saturday, and food prep for the week on Sunday, you will be able to enjoy their company more often while staying on track.

This is also where giving fit back comes into play. You can lead, influence, and create opportunities for your friends, helping them embark on their own fitness journey. We know that just because we make better choices and adjust our lifestyle, others around us may not follow suit. In part, this is a cultural ritual. Every January, when people have made their New Year's resolutions, many are on a new diet or weight-loss craze, that unlike RedeFit, are not lifestyle programs. Inevitably by March, most have reverted to their old habits. So, when a friend is making lifestyle changes, we will be supportive but have a wait-and-see perspective. By living the lean, happy, healthy lifestyle, your friends will see the sustainability and your happiness. Like anything worthwhile, giving fit back is a process and not a short-term endeavor.

Giving fit back only requires that you share your strengths, challenges, perseverance, and willingness to learn along the way.

GFB TO YOUR COMMUNITY

We've repeatedly talked about the tribe mentality, and in giving fit back to your community. We will discuss leading and influencing your tribe or joining an existing one that supports your journey. The choices under this category are only limited by your creativity, but it can be helpful to think of them as three options.

The first option is to offer your time or resources to an existing organization. Examples include volunteering at a soup kitchen, donating time and resources to a healthy school lunch program or a program that provides weekend meals for low-income children or volunteering at a 5K race to support runners. These are just a few ideas for you to positively impact the fitness journey of those around you.

Another option is to start something new, such as launching a run club. Initially, this may sound overwhelming, and you may feel that you need to be an expert. In practice, it's simple. For example, you could create a Facebook page or even just post an announcement about new runners getting together. Just set the date and time and show up. You could even tag some friends to make sure they see your post. You never know who will show up; you might interest just one person, or you might attract 20 people. No matter what the outcome, you've made it easier for others and yourself to be consistent with your fitness journey. You've given fit back.

The third option is guiding people one-on-one. Again, expertise is not required; the only thing required is living the fit lifestyle and being empathetic to others' unique journeys. An example is sharing with your fitness buddy the difference between commercial smoothies loaded with sugar and calories and healthy ones they can easily make at home. It can be as simple as sharing the strategies you've used for eating healthily on busy work days.

When people can see that you're experiencing the same struggles, are facing the same obstacles, and have found a way to be successful, you'll have a wonderful opportunity to provide them with the tools to succeed on their journey.

None of the above options is better than the others. Your offers to assist can be large or small. Offering to regularly walk with someone who wants to improve their daily endurance is as powerful as a larger-scale endeavor. The focus is on improving the community. Pick an area of the RedeFit Model in which you excel and help others in that area or select an area you struggle with and count on group support to help you reach your goals.

Don't be afraid to think outside the box and be an initiator. This can be difficult at first, but with a little effort, you can greatly influence your community and yourself to achieve the fit lifestyle. Even if you impact just one person, you are giving fit back.

GFB REINFORCES YOUR OWN FITNESS.

One of the best parts of your family, friends, co-workers, and community living a fit lifestyle is that it becomes much easier for you to do the same. Take a moment to consider your life of fitness with others on the same path. Imagine family dinners where great tasting and healthy food is served. Imagine friends inviting you on a hike capped off by wine tasting at a winery. Imagine a birthday celebration focused on fun activities with people you enjoy as opposed to making sweet cake loaded with frosting as the main activity. You'd have a blast and wouldn't even miss the sugar high, which is inevitably followed by a crash. The goal isn't to deprive yourself; the goal is to enjoy life to the fullest while also living a fit lifestyle. When you encourage others to choose the fit lifestyle, it reinforces your belief in it, which will help you stay on track.

GFB HAS A RIPPLE EFFECT TO MAKE THE WORLD A BETTER PLACE.

The beauty of the RedeFit approach is that we are not encouraging people to get fit solely to improve their appearance. Our approach results in healthier, more mindful people with better relationships, and a greater sense of community. Isn't that the world we would like to live in? It starts with just one person—you. The ripple effect of your daily actions has the power to influence the world now and for many generations to come. Live the life you've always dreamed of—active, healthy, engaged, and inspired.

The table below presents recommendations for giving fit back. In the ADD column, we propose behaviors to add to your daily activities. In the LIMIT column, we include behaviors to limit in your daily activities.

ADD
Recognize that you're an influencer.
Cook a healthy meal for a friend or a family member.
Compliment others trying to improve their fitness.
LIMIT
Avoid justifying yourself to others.
Stop being hard on yourself for not being perfect.
Don't participate in activities with others that are inconsistent with your fitness goals.

For a deeper understanding of these and other strategies, visit TheRedefit.com

----

We all have our own biases, but the more careful we are to guide people to their personal niche and favorite tools and tricks, the more we are truly giving fit back.

NOTES FROM THE DOC

For most people, thinking about giving fit back, or leading by example, can feel daunting. We may not see ourselves as leaders capable of making an impact, especially in an area we're still working on. Similarly, in our culture of excess, as we commit to a fit lifestyle, it may feel like we are in the minority. What is the likelihood that those in the minority can impact those in the majority? Contrary to popular belief, it's highly likely. In social psychology, this is called conversion theory. Research suggests that a consistent minority can exert as much of an influence as a consistent majority, and even more notable, the minority will likely have a greater effect on a deeper level because they impact belief systems. This happens through five key influences: 1) The minority exhibits consistent behavior; 2) Possessing confidence in the face of social pressure; 3) The change happens through change of perspectives (not just compliance); 4) The more the minority challenges and engages with previous perspectives, the more significant the conversion and 5) Others identify with those in the minority.

Consistency is not about perfection, but a consistent theme running through your words and actions over time.

CONSISTENCY

The first of the key influences that impacts conversion is consistency. Wait, don't tune out yet. I know consistency is the bane of most people's lives. It's basically a compound four-letter word that describes why and how we fall off our wagons. It does not mean you have to do everything perfectly. It means you must have a consistent message and actions that people can count on. For example, I told my boys repeatedly growing up (they are now young men) that too much sugar is bad—empty calories, energy dip, and hard on the teeth). However, they have seen me eat dessert and enjoy a soda. Sounds inconsistent—right? Not really, because they have also seen me make choices throughout the week to balance sugar with healthier choices. When they lived at home and I prepared healthy meals, their response was often an eye-roll or a grunt (okay, I still get those). However, now when my college-aged son comes home for a meal and I offer him his favorite sweet snack, he will decline and say he had enough sugar and needs to cut back. *Did he really say that?* My youngest reads drink labels and compare sugar levels. He might argue with me if I say something else would be better. He sometimes proves me wrong. I don't always eat perfectly or avoid temptations, but my message and actions of moderation and awareness are consistent and have clearly made an impact.

CONFIDENCE

Conversion also requires confidence in the face of social pressure. My boys don't always appreciate my educational nuggets about regular exercise and good nutrition. My friends have ribbed me about turning down a second cocktail or fast food, and coworkers have given me unflattering nicknames, implying that I am no fun.

Most of us have experienced this for our healthy choices. But if we stay the course and are not impacted by social pressure and criticism, our children will model our behaviors and friends will ask for advice on things like choosing the best yoga studio or making healthy choices when eating out. It's easy to cave to peer pressure and sometimes you will. Positive self-talk and finding a tribe that supports you when you are struggling are key to a consistent message and remaining confident.

UNBIASED

For consistency to have an impact, your behavior must appear unbiased. When we educate ourselves on the rationale behind our health and fitness choices, our minority voice holds enormous weight. You have undoubtedly observed your friends or family embracing the latest workout craze. They may urge you to join them because they claim it's amazing; in fact, they sometimes border on zealousness. So, why don't you join them? Probably because you have been down that road before. Their new diet or workout craze lasts maybe a month or two and then they move on to the next fad. We're all guilty of it to some degree.

I recently bought a fancy new water bottle to remind me to stay hydrated. Will this luring technology do the trick? Or is my latest solution not enough? I don't know how long my water bottle kick is going to last, but I do not plan to sing its praises on social media. Why not? Because when you zealously proclaim that you have discovered a panacea to all health issues—like drinking enough water—it screams compliance with the majority bias—the hot ticket of the day. It reveals that you are not on a targeted journey but rather following the social tide.

My fitness routine is mostly weight training and yoga. I invite friends to go with me, but I also encourage whatever they are doing, such as walking or playing tennis. I know that regular exercise that works for their lifestyle and body is important, not my newest passion. When people ask me what I eat, I tell them, but I emphasize my thinking about nutrition, not key foods they must eat. I highlight my ongoing trial and error and offer resources, including experts, I have used. We all have our own biases, but the more careful we are to guide people to their personal niche and favorite tools and tricks, the more we are truly giving fit back.

ENGAGEMENT

Another key factor for conversion, as opposed to compliance, is to actively engage others with what you are doing and thinking. This means having discussions, showing by example and even challenging each other. Pairing writing with auditory or visual learning helps us to learn more effectively. Practicing something like tennis or yoga helps with muscle memory and more consistent success. The same is true when we are learning new concepts and challenging our previous mindset. If someone tells us to try hot yoga or replace Cheetos with kale chips just because we should, how likely are we to stick with it? So, when someone challenges that their lack of flexibility makes hot yoga impossible, the answer should not be: "Suck it up. You will be fine." Instead, we educate and encourage. We engage in what they are concerned about. We acknowledge poor flexibility is a real thing. We share examples of our own flexibility journey and facts like 200lb+ football players are doing it as part of their team workouts for that very reason. Flexibility is accessible for everyone and prevents injuries.

When someone argues that kale chips are not their thing, engagement means we can ask questions about their taste preferences (sweet or savory for example) and suggest other snacks that are healthier, then sample some together. Humans learn by exploring, breaking things down, debating, and trying. The RedeFit Model was developed for this very reason. We are giving you the information you need to explore your needs and the various tools that match your lifestyle and stage on your fitness journey. Those around you will benefit from the same approach as you share what you learn.

IDENTIFICATION

One of the greatest misconceptions is that you must be really together and incredibly fit to give fit back and positively influence others. Social psychology challenges this theory. People identify with others like them. We connect based on things like gender, age, height, culture, occupation, and interests. There is comfort in knowing that someone relates to what you consider important and what you find hard. We want to learn from each other. Getting fit is no different.

As I mentioned previously, I am working to learn how to do handstands properly. I tried to learn this once before when I was still in schools. However, long, lanky girls like me were discouraged from participating in sports like gymnastics. In fact, I was kicked out of a gymnastics program because the coach said I was too tall and would never get it. That stayed with me for a long time.

In recent years, several acquaintances, both taller and larger, were making great progress with handstands. Their challenges were like mine. Seeing how hard they worked—that it was neither easy nor flawless—encouraged me to try harder, even though I frequently failed. They are giving fit back just by sharing their journey—one that I wanted to be on with them.

In the world of highlight reels on social media, it's important to not get caught up in the skewed personas people project and to remember who we are. Our struggles and efforts are so much more important than a perfect outcome. Giving fit back only requires that you share your strengths, challenges, perseverance, and willingness to learn along the way.

Footnotes

Chapter 1: The Broken Fitness Industry
1) Jack Zenger and Joseph Folkman, "The Ideal Praise to Criticism Ratio," *Harvard Business Review*, (2013), https://hbr.org/2013/03/the-ideal-praise-to-criticism.

2) Allison Wood Brooks, "Get Excited: Reappraising Pre-Performance Anxiety as Excitement," *Journal of Psychology*, Vol. 143, No. 3, (2013): pp. 1144 –1158 0096-3445/14/ DOI: 10.1037/a0035325

Chapter 2: Creating the Habit of Consistency
1) J Coates, *The Hour Between Dog and Wolf: Risk Taking, Gut Feelings and the Biology of Boom and Bust.* (New York: Penguin Books, 2012).

2) Samuele Zilioli, Neil V. Watson, "Testosterone Across Successive Competitions: Evidence for a 'Winner Effect' in Humans?" Behavioral Endocrinology Laboratory, Department of Psychology, Simon Fraser University, *Canada Psychoneuroendocrinology* 47 (2014): 1—9.

3) Tiziana Zalla et al., "Differential Amygdala Responses to Winning and Losing: a Functional Magnetic Resonance Imaging Study in Humans," *European Journal of Neuroscience*, First published: December 24, 2001, https://doi.org/10.1046/j.1460-9568.2000.00064.x.

4) Albert Bandura, "Six Theories of Child Development, Social Cognitive Theory," In R. Vasta (Ed.), *Annals of Child Development*. Vol. 6 (1989): 1-60. Greenwich, CT: JAI Press.
Albert Bandura, "The Power of Observational Learning Through Social Modeling."
Robert Sternberg et al. *Scientists Making a Difference* (Cambridge: Cambridge University Press, 2016), pp. 235-239.

5) Edward M. Robertson, Alvaro Pascual-Leone, Chris Miall, "Current Concepts in Procedural Consolidation," *Nature Reviews Neuroscience,* 5 (2004): 576—582.

6) Daryl B. O'Connor et al. "Activational Effects of Testosterone on Cognitive Function in Men," *Neuropsychologia* 39 (2001): 1385—1394.

Chapter 3: The RedeFit Model
1) Gary P. Latham, "Goal-Setting Theory: Causal Relationships, Mediators, and Moderators," *Oxford Research Encyclopedia of Psychology*, Online Publication Date: May 2016, DOI: 10.1093/acrefore/9780190236557.013.12

2) Daniel Kahneman, *Thinking Fast and Slow* (New York: Farrar, Straus and Giroux, 2011)

3) Esther K. Papies, "Goal Priming as a Situated Intervention Tool," *Current Opinion in Psychology,* Volume 12 (2016): pp. 12-16.

Chapter 4: Mindset
1) Carol S. Dweck, *Mindset: The New Psychology of Success* (New York: Ballantine Books, 2008).

Chapter 5: Stress
1) Norman B. Anderson, PhD, Cynthia D. Belar, PhD, et al., "Stress in America: Paying With Our Health, February 4, 2015, https://www.apa.org/news/press/releases/stress/2014/stress-report.pdf.

2) Bruce McEwen, Carla Nasca, et al. "Stress-induced Structural Plasticity of Medial Amygdala Stellate Neurons and Rapid Prevention by a Candidate Antidepressant," *Molecular Psychiatry* (2016) DOI: 10.1038/MP.2016.68.

3) Robert Epstein, "How Best to Fight Stress: Measuring and Ranking Relevant Competencies," Paper presented at the 91st annual meeting of the Western Psychological Association, Los Angeles, CA, April 2011.

Chapter 8: Nutrition
1) John D. Eastwood et al. "The Unengaged Mind: Defining Boredom in Terms of Attention." *Perspectives in Psychological Science* Volume: 7 issue (2012): 482-495.

2) Leo Widrich, "Why We Have Our Best Ideas in the Shower," Buffer.com, last modified September 7, 2018, https://blog.bufferapp.com/why-we-have-our-best-ideas-in-the-shower-the-science-of-creativity

3) Karen L. Swartz, M.D. "Origins of Depression," Remedies: Health Communities.com, last modified August 16, 2013, http://www.healthcommunities.com/depression/origins-of-depression_jhmwp.shtml.

45861974R00116

Made in the USA
Lexington, KY
21 July 2019